Overcoming Infertility

A CLEVELAND CLINIC GUIDE

Tommaso Falcone, M.D.

with Davis Young

OVERCOMING INFERTILITY
A CLEVELAND CLINIC GUIDE

Cleveland Clinic Press/May 2006
All rights reserved
Copyright © The Cleveland Clinic Foundation

Contact:

Cleveland Clinic Press

9500 Euclid Ave. NA32

Cleveland, OH 44195

216-444-1158

chilnil@ccf.org

www.clevelandclinicpress.org

This book is not intended to replace personal medical care and supervision; there is no substitute for the experience and information that your doctor can provide. Rather, it is our hope that this book will provide additional information to help people understand the nature and diagnosis of infertility.

Proper medical care should always be tailored to the individual patient. If you read something in this book that seems to conflict with your doctor's instructions, contact your doctor. Since each individual case differs, there will be good reasons for individual treatment to differ from the information presented in this book.

If you have any questions about any treatment in this book, consult your doctor.

The patient names and cases used in this book do not represent actual people, but are composite cases drawn from several sources.

ISBN: 1596240245

Falcone, Tommaso.

Overcoming infertility: A Cleveland Clinic Guide/Tommaso Falcone with Davis Young.

p. cm.

1. Infertility–Popular works. 2. Infertility–Treatment–Popular works.

3. Human reproductive technology–Popular works. I. Young, Davis, 1939-II. Cleveland Clinic. III. Title.

RC889.F353 2006   616.6'9206–dc22
                    2006008155

Cover and Book Design: Whitney Campbell & Co. • Advertising & Design

Illustrations by Joseph Kanasz, BFA

Contents

Introduction

"Everybody lives for something better to come."

– Anonymous

"I got my hands on every infertility book I could find. I borrowed some. I bought some. I found them to be very negative about things like medication side effects and hyper-stimulation syndrome. All those books did was scare me. In fact, for two or three years after that, I was so scared from reading those books that I did nothing.

"I hope this book is very positive. I would like people to know they shouldn't listen to the horror stories of other people. Just go into your treatment with a very positive outlook. I think if you're very positive about it and you work hard enough at it that you will probably get children. Medicine has come so far now that almost anything can be overcome."

Those are the words of one of our patients and her reaction to the challenge of infertility treatments.

She sought information. Some of what she found was probably pretty good. Without a doubt, she came across some misinformation as well. She was troubled by the tone of much of what she read. She became confused and frightened. As a result, she let time elapse. And during this period when she took no action, her feelings of frustration, disappointment, and anger over not being a mom did nothing but magnify.

This was not a happy time in her life. Fortunately, she ultimately made the journey to parenthood. It was not easy, but she persevered.

With infertility – as with all of medicine – there is no cookie-cutter experience. Somehow, an egg and a sperm have to come from different directions to find each other and become one. Every situation is unique. Some patients tolerate pain well; others don't. Some handle the emotional stresses of infertility well; others find them more difficult. Some get great results; some do not.

In many instances, there's some sort of problem that prevents an egg or a sperm from even starting the journey. In other cases, the journey may be started, but it cannot be completed. And there are times when an egg and a sperm actually do get "eyeball to eyeball," so to speak, but still no connection is made.

There are many reasons (and combinations of reasons) why getting pregnant just doesn't work for some people. When that happens, there are three basic options:

1. Give up.

2. Stay hopeful and keep trying your way.

3. Channel your hope and seek professional help.

This is a book for people who choose the third option – for people who have come to a point in their lives where they remain hopeful and are prepared to reach out for the professional help they need to be successful. This is a book for people who are ready to move forward with medical treatment of their infertility.

This book doesn't pretend to hold every answer. Nor does it address in great detail every possible scenario. If it did, it would be a medical textbook or maybe even a series of medical textbooks. Rather, this is a *consumer* guide to infertility issues. The intent is to provide the essential information you will need to either (1) start making good choices or (2) whet your appetite to subsequently seek even more information from the many good sources available.

Everyone associated with our practice wants you to find hope, but we don't want you to experience false hope. So this book is intended to be a blend of hope and reality.

The techniques to treat infertility and the outcomes of those treatments improve all the time. That is undeniably true. But the treatment of infertility is still a long way from producing the same results for everyone. Anybody who tells you differently is wrong. There is nothing automatic about addressing infertility issues.

Infertility treatment combines good science with the art of adapting to the individual circumstances of each patient. Many people have a good chance. Nobody has a guarantee. That is the blend of hope and reality this book tries to present.

Because we have dealt with so many patients, it has become increasingly clear to us over time that a need exists to further demystify the challenge of overcoming infertility. Yes, it can be complex. But it is not so complex that it cannot be understood. There is virtually no end to scientific papers and books on infertility for medical professionals. On the other hand, there is always room for good information for patients – information that strikes that right balance between hope and reality.

You will see that we have started each chapter with a quotation that is positive and hopeful. These are taken from *The Book of Positive Quotations* (compiled and arranged by John Cook and published by Fairview Press).

We go on to provide basic explanations, overviews, and summaries about infertility and its treatments. Detailed information is included in sections titled "Medically speaking." And if you want to dig into the subject even further, we have listed numerous credible resources in Chapter 12. This book is organized in a way that facilitates further investigation at whatever level is appropriate for you.

We have included a number of patient experiences as well. Some have ended with a happier result than others. We would be less than honest if we did not acknowledge that and present a range of experiences, including those of married couples, a single-sex couple, and a single mom. We are deeply indebted to these patients who shared their stories so that you can learn from them, and we hope their stories will help to keep your spirits up.

Some patients can be treated at relatively low levels of infertility medicine. The cases we have highlighted in this book all required more than that. On the far end of the spectrum is the story of a couple who failed at every attempt to conceive, but who are now the proud and happy parents of two adopted children.

Some families had one child; some had more. Some had twins who are separated in age because a frozen embryo was retrieved at a later date. One had triplets. Every story is real. Every story is different. Every story is compelling.

Along the way, these patients handled the physical and emotional pain differently. The expression "no pain, no gain" is the reality of infertility treatment. We always "hope" there is no pain. The "reality" is that there is almost always some pain. That is just the way it is.

If these patient experiences are so different, is there anything that binds these folks together?

Yes.

They all knew what they wanted. The goal was clear in every case: a baby. They were all committed to achieving their goal – one way or another. Long before they ever reached our doorstep, many had been to other doctors, experienced numerous tests, and tried a wide range of remedies.

Nobody starts with an infertility specialist. You get to us after dealing with an OB/GYN and often at the referral of that doctor. And, in many cases, patients find their way to us after having first worked with another specialist.

Patients who come our way have been frustrated by their failure to create a baby. They are upset when we first see them. There are no exceptions. All of those featured in this book were able to pick themselves up and keep going. They had their hopes challenged, but none ever lost hope. That recurrent feeling of hope is what inspired them to come to us in the first place. They may have been frustrated and upset, but they were not hopeless. And we believe they would all tell you they are stronger today for having gone through the experience, regardless of how their individual journey ended.

Now, let's focus on you.

By the time you get to an infertility specialist, it is highly likely that there will be no quick fix or easy answer. You are opening yourself and, in most cases, your spouse to a process that will take some time. It's important to learn patience, and one way to achieve that state is to become an informed medical consumer. The intent of this book is to help you do that.

As you begin your own challenging journey, my associates and I sincerely hope you have a positive experience with a good ending.

Tommaso Falcone, M.D.

Chairman, Department of Obstetrics & Gynecology

Cleveland Clinic

Chapter 1
You Are Not Alone!

> *"Nothing happens unless first a dream."*
>
> *– Carl Sandburg*

You have been trying for some time – without success – to get pregnant. This has made you exceedingly sad. You are not alone!

You think it's your fault. You are blaming yourself, and you feel guilty about dragging your spouse into what you think is your issue. You are concerned that this may be harming your relationship.

You think if you just keep trying longer, something good may happen. You know you are a good person and strongly believe you deserve to be a parent.

You probably have been to other doctors. You've undergone a variety of testing and perhaps some treatments, and you've incurred expense. There have been no solutions. This is very disappointing.

Your spouse may not be as supportive as you would like. His or her focus on this issue does not match yours. Or your other half may in fact be totally engaged in the issue, but nobody can tell either of you why you're not getting pregnant. You are not receiving answers, and this is enormously frustrating.

Your health insurance does not cover infertility treatments. There are house payments and car payments and credit card debts, and you worry about how you will ever be able to afford infertility treatments. You know there are no guarantees, and that makes it hard for you to justify either the effort or the expense. If you are miserable now, how miserable will you be if you get to the end of the line and fail?

You get scared when you think of the possibility of multiple births. That would be extremely difficult. On the other hand, you want children so badly. You go back and forth on this issue.

You think about what you will do if you end up with unused embryos. You worry about the ethical ramifications of what you might choose.

You need somebody to talk to, but perhaps you are from a family that doesn't listen or you know your family members would not be supportive even if they did listen. You don't know whom to tell or how much to tell them.

You think about how you will react and how your spouse will react if there is a need for a sperm donor or a surrogate – or both.

You are conflicted about whether to embrace high-tech treatment. You tell yourself that what your infertility specialist has to offer is neither natural nor spontaneous. You find it is a hard concept to get your mind around.

You are upset a lot. This issue is dominating your life. You are still hopeful, but each day it becomes harder for you to sustain that hope.

You are depressed. Life isn't as much fun as it used to be. Your friends have children and you don't. It simply destroys you emotionally to go to a baby shower for somebody else.

You don't know where to turn for solid, factual information. So you turn everywhere. You get conflicting signals. You turn off. But you are not alone!

Emphatically, you are not alone!

As lonely as you may feel at this very moment, you are not alone.

The first step in addressing your infertility issues is for you to accept the fact that you are not alone. Somewhere out there is support for you. Do all you can to find it.

The challenge of your lifetime

As you already know, creating a baby isn't always easy. Many people find it can be very difficult. Unfortunately, you are one of those people.

What should be a happy pursuit has instead become an endurance test. It is like running a distance race. If you can cross the finish line, the effort to get there is well worth it.

In the process of analyzing your infertility issues, there certainly will be tests and perhaps some combination of drug therapy and surgical procedures. In contemplating that prospect, you might want to keep in mind the words of the patient cited in the book's introduction: "Just go into your treatment with a very positive outlook."

Every bit of whatever you are about to experience involves science – perhaps some of it extremely high-tech. In recent years, this high-tech science has brought about many enhancements in infertility treatments. These advances have improved outcomes significantly. There is real forward momentum in the field of assisted reproductive technology (ART), and this trend will continue in the future at an accelerated pace. That is assured.

But as with many fields of medicine – and particularly with respect to infertility and the undeniable excellence of the scientific effort that is going into this field – success will always continue to depend on more than just technology.

The success you want so much can be elusive, and it can involve a journey that includes many twists and turns. Commitment, perseverance, and confidence are not scientific matters. These are matters of the spirit – your spirit. They must be considered in combination with the science of infertility.

We call that type of approach treating the whole person. This is the standard you should expect from any leading infertility practice: good science and good people skills that address your condition broadly, not narrowly.

The right approach to infertility is one that treats the body, mind, and spirit.

Understanding your infertility

We are no longer surprised when patients like you come for your first visit and it is apparent you have done a lot of advance homework. Why wouldn't you? You are probably facing life-changing decisions. What could be more important than that?

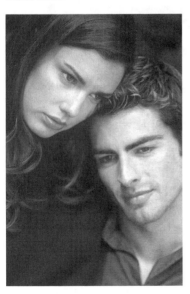

Wherever you may have turned for information in your journey so far, the important message to us is that you clearly want to learn more and remain actively involved in the decision-making process with respect to your own case. It is incumbent upon us as medical professionals to facilitate that involvement for you.

From the moment we first meet, we need to understand each other. That means those of us who are on the treatment side of the relationship must be clear, direct, and understandable. We must always speak in ways that communicate instead of intimidate.

Beyond that, each of us needs to actively listen. Each of us needs to ask thoughtful questions. Each of us needs to provide accurate responses.

Sometimes I think the term infertility specialist is actually a misnomer. What we are really all about is helping people become fertile. That is an important distinction. Everything we do has the objective of helping you have a baby. Your goal is our goal.

In the final analysis, there is only one way a baby is created – a sperm and an egg unite. There is no other way. That has never changed. What has changed are the new ways that can happen. Today, there are more and better ways to achieve fertility than at any former time. If you choose to become involved in a fertility program, you will confront choices in how to help that sperm and egg get together. Some of these choices were not available just a few years ago. It is important to understand those choices, and it is essential to make good ones.

Information and hope are the building blocks of good choices. And good choices increase your chances of reaching the finish line.

Turning "scare" into "care"

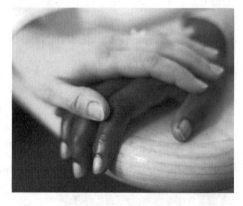

Fear is often cited as a great motivator. Fear of being fired, for example, may cause you to change how you interact with others in the workplace. Fear of disappointing a relative or friend can inspire you to alter a negative behavior pattern and improve relationships in the process.

Healthy fear can be your friend, but unhealthy fear can be a great intimidator. Unhealthy fear is often present when people are asked to deal with the unknown. For any first-time patient, infertility represents the unknown.

We acknowledge that infertility issues can be scary for people. Regardless of any advance homework you do before reaching us, you are still dealing largely with the unknown unless you have previously been through an infertility program. So if you are new to all of this, it can be intimidating. It is important for you to know that most specialists who deal with infertility issues are sensitive to that.

Perhaps you have never thought about infertility issues until recently and you have a lot of concerns. The job of an infertility practice is to help you deal with each concern in the process of helping you to understand your infertility.

First of all, it's important to put it into perspective. Although this book is for and about you, infertility problems are widespread. Many people are in your shoes.

In recent years, there appears to have been an increase in infertility rates in the so-called developed countries, including the United States. Why is that? Several factors seem to be in play. One is that there is simply more awareness of infertility by the general public. The issue is being addressed more often and in more settings than ever before. This is a good thing.

A second is a surge in the rate of sexually transmitted diseases, which can be so devastating to fertility. At a minimum, STDs are often a major obstacle to fertility. Sadly, in some cases, they can permanently prevent fertility.

A third is that people are waiting longer to have children – in many cases too long. Much has been written about how people are postponing families – often for too long from a pregnancy perspective. One woman in five today is having her first child after the age of 35.

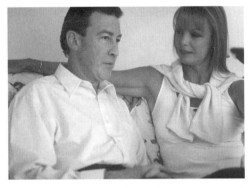

Age is a serious challenge. As a woman's age goes up, her fertility potential goes down. This is never a good thing. This is not to pressure you into having children before you are ready, but rather to simply inform you that age can be a very complicating factor.

The medical community is in general agreement that couples may have infertility issues if there are no results after one year of trying to achieve pregnancy. If you are a woman in your mid-30s, you should not wait even a year before seeking a fertility evaluation.

In general terms, at about age 37 or 38, a woman's opportunity to conceive and to have a full-term successful pregnancy begins to diminish quickly and dramatically. What we might have been able to treat at a younger age with drug therapy or a basic surgical procedure now might require a much more exotic and expensive approach. And the odds of achieving your goal are reduced the older you become, regardless of the process or how much money you are willing to spend.

One of our nurses put it well when she said it is heartbreaking to see patients who could have been helped if only they had come to us at a younger age.

If you want to be parents, please be careful that you do not wait too long. People often refer to the fact that, for a woman, the biological clock is ticking. That really is true. Everything about a woman's reproductive system is different at 27 than it is at 37. We can do a lot for you, but we cannot make you 27 again. Neither can we make you 32 again.

Infertility by the numbers

It is generally believed that about 6 million women in the United States have an infertility issue, with somewhere between 2 million and 3 million receiving counseling, testing, or treatment.

Big numbers like 6 million or even 2 million are hard to grasp. Few of us can put those numbers into the context of our daily lives.

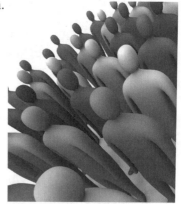

The more widespread the geography, the bigger the numbers become. If there are 6 million American women with infertility problems, there are many more than 6 million with the same issues on a global basis.

But suppose we were to tell you that of every one hundred people of prime childbearing age walking down the street, ten to fifteen of them have an infertility issue? Think about it. That is a lot of people. Any of us can understand the numbers when put in that context – ten to fifteen of every one hundred of child-bearing age.

Look at the numbers from another perspective. Visualize a neighborhood with one hundred homes. Suppose in that particular neighborhood there is an infertility issue in each of those homes. In perhaps forty, the woman will have the issue. In another ten, the man has it. In forty more, both the man and the woman have infertility issues. What about the other ten houses? They have what we call unexplained infertility. Does that mean they will never have a child? No. What it does mean is that after extensive testing, the cause of infertility cannot be identified. And, in fact, it may never be identified.

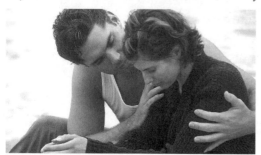

We can understand numbers when they are presented like that. And we can also begin to understand why infertility is often referred to as a "couple's problem." It is indeed a couple's problem for two key reasons:

1. Lots of men have problems that contribute to infertility.

2. Couples need to approach infertility as "our problem," not "your problem," or they may not remain couples.

Let's look at the numbers from yet another perspective. If the residents of all one hundred homes entered into a good infertility program, how many would someday go home with a baby? For that question, there is no one answer. It depends on many factors. The question you ultimately want to ask is this: For people my age with my issue, what are my chances? Keep that question in mind. You will want to ask it.

Not everyone succeeds quickly. Some do not succeed at all. But nobody succeeds without trying. Based on your situation, you have to decide how committed you are to participating in an infertility program.

Or to put it another way, are you willing to risk failure in the pursuit of success?

"Why me?"

This is a common question. It may be a fair question, but we think the better question is simply: "Why?"

That is what we need to figure out – together. Maximizing fertility potential is a job for a highly trained team dedicated to that specialty. When you enter an infertility program, that team becomes your team.

Whatever your issue, a major infertility practice should be able to address it from the standpoint of experience. It is hard to imagine any fertility-preventing problem that such a practice has not seen before – many times. This does not mean the staff will take a calloused view of your issue. It should mean the doctors and other health-care professionals will help you address your issue with a reassuring combination of understanding and experience.

Fixing fertility issues starts when you take ownership of your issues. Medical professionals can help address them, but in the final analysis, you will own the problem, solution, and result. The first step to taking ownership is to want and accept that ownership.

It is useful to reconsider the analogy of the distance runner. Running is often thought of as a solitary pursuit. You will find that in many respects, participating in an infertility program can also be a lonely endeavor. You may have a great spouse or partner, but there will be plenty of times when you are alone with your feelings and your fears. But if you are an elite runner – or if you choose to become a dedicated patient – you will be surrounded by a support team focused on helping you win.

With runners, it is all about equipment selection, treatment of old injuries, eating smart, strength, and conditioning. Those issues get a lot of focus. What might appear to be a lonely pursuit is really a team effort designed to help maximize running potential.

That is exactly the approach of a good infertility practice. We are in the business of helping maximize your fertility potential. It takes a team approach. It is about compiling the right information. It is about technical execution. It is about helping you stay focused on the goal. It is about balancing hope and reality.

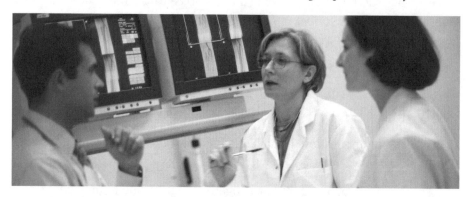

All of that requires highly trained people with complementary skill sets.

- A medical team that understands the challenge. Experience really is the best teacher.

- A medical team that believes good communication with each other and with you is central to success. This means a team that knows how to listen and also knows how to talk clearly with patients.

- A medical team that knows success is built on executing every small step well, not just the big ones. You can reach your goal – a baby – only with good execution by both you and your medical team. You have to pay close attention to all of the details along the way.

- A medical team committed to your goal. As people often say, "Keep your eyes on the prize."

It really is your goal. You really will own that goal. But you can have a lot of support if you are open to it. That includes support by your medical team. If you make good choices along the way, you can have a great medical team working with you to achieve your goal.

Summary

Many people have infertility issues. Addressing them is not always easy, pleasant, or inexpensive. But people who focus on the goal versus the process will almost always say they would do it all again.

Never forget this: You are not alone!

Let's get started

In the pages that follow, we will be looking at these key issues:

- Finding good information and choosing the right infertility specialist. This is not a task to be approached in a casual way.

- Doing all you can to prevent infertility from happening to you. Whatever happens, don't be your own worst enemy.

- Identifying infertility issues in both women and men. The difficulty can be with either one of you. It can be both of you. It is critical to determine that and deal with the issues.

- Range of treatment options from the most basic to the most sophisticated. You want to be in the hands of an infertility practice that offers all of the options.

- Touchy ethical and religious issues: single parents, cancer, accidents, genetic testing, selective reduction, donor programs, and more. The first step in dealing with the touchy issues is to acknowledge they exist.

- Costs. You need to go into this with your eyes wide open.

- Gaining and keeping control of your emotions. Infertility treatment is often described as an emotional roller coaster. We want to make sure you have your seat belt fastened.

- Hanging tough when things don't always go your way. You will find that perseverance goes hand in hand with success.

- Additional information resources available to you. We will point you in the right direction.

- A glossary of terms that will help demystify some of the confusing medical and infertility lingo.

In looking at these issues, we will include:

- "Plain talk" chapter overviews about each major subject.

- "Medically speaking" sections, which provide a more in-depth look at medical issues.

- Frequently asked questions. We also will suggest some questions you should be asking yourself.

- "Front-line perspectives" from some of the people delivering care at our infertility practice.

- "Patient talk" – real patients' experiences in their own words.

- Definitions of key terms – not too many, but the key ones.

It is now time to get started. That begins with gathering information and choosing a doctor.

Chapter 2

Getting Information and Choosing Your Infertility Specialist

"More powerful than the will to win is the courage to begin."

– Anonymous

You have tried to get pregnant for some time. Month after month, you have experienced tremendous hope only to confront a harsh and unpleasant reality. The time has come to bundle up all the anger, disappointment, and sadness and turn that energy into positive action.

You are ready to get serious about gathering information. You are ready to get serious about selecting an infertility specialist.

So where do you turn? How do you get started?

A great deal of information about infertility is easily accessible in many forms. The Internet has some outstanding websites devoted to infertility issues. It also has some websites that are not so terrific. It's important to be careful.

Numerous books show up when you Google retail bookstore sites. There are videotapes. There are audiotapes. And there are brochures put out by individual infertility practices, hospitals, professional associations, and providers of goods and services to the infertility marketplace. If you look around, you will probably be able to find informational seminars as well.

Finally, you may have friends and acquaintances who have been through what you are about to go through. In many cases, they will be happy to share those experiences.

So the quantity of information and its availability are not an issue. The issue is the quality of that information.

Something else that matters is, of course, the ability of an individual patient – especially somebody new to infertility treatment – to be able to know the difference between bad information and good information, and to reject what isn't good. It is often difficult for somebody to be able to make fact-based choices versus emotion-based choices. Haven't we all been in situations where our emotions overwhelm our better instincts?

Always remember, you are in charge. Part of being in charge – a very important part – relates to good initial choices. In this instance, that means doing the homework to find both the right information resources and the right medical resources.

Getting information

Here, we'll inject a cautionary note: Look at all information very carefully. One of the best resources is the American Society for Reproductive Medicine. ASRM has done an excellent job of translating the complexities of infertility into an easily understood format. It offers helpful information on its website (www.asrm.org) and provides a number of consumer-friendly pamphlets. It also can help you find a doctor.

Professional society websites have been reviewed by medical people who consider the information provided on them to be credible. There are many sources, particularly on the Internet, that do not measure up to the accuracy of information provided by an organization such as ASRM. For example, the information in Internet chat rooms is not all bad, but certainly there is enough in that category to cause considerable concern. It is not at all unusual for us to start a new patient relationship by correcting opinions based on misinformation.

Something else to beware of is tabloid journalism about celebrity pregnancies. Often what those reports fail to mention is that the 40-plus celebrity mom had to use a surrogate and perhaps also needed donor eggs. There is no magic potion for celebrities who are over 40. Their eggs get old just like anybody else's. The media reports that fail to mention this do a disservice to people like you.

Here's another cautionary note: Friends who want to be helpful often aren't when it comes to talking about their medical experiences. This is not because they have bad motives. Rather, in their zeal to be helpful, they can go over the line in terms of presenting opinions as absolute facts. If your well-intentioned friends tell you something that doesn't sound right, chances are it's not. Somewhere between friends wanting to offer encouragement and others unknowingly terrifying you, the truth can be found. As with most things in life, the truth is usually found in the middle.

Always check with medical professionals before you accept as gospel the opinions of nonmedical people. Where your friends (and family) can be most helpful is in listening to you and being unconditionally supportive. Rely on them for that. Rely on organizations such as ASRM and on professionals like your doctor for the unvarnished, unemotional facts about infertility.

Among other resources for the high-quality information you need are books by recognized professionals in the field. But train yourself to step back and take a hard look at what you read. Treating infertility is never about magic. We all love a good magician, but in this case, what you need is a good doctor. Some books are better than others.

Determining the accuracy of information

Let me give you a little medical background that may be helpful as you find and evaluate information. This will point out the potential pitfalls in accepting information at face value.

Doctors today offer recommendations founded on what is called "evidence-based medicine." This is widely considered the ideal approach to medical care. In the past, much of medicine was based primarily on the experience of earlier practitioners and on observation. Opinions offered by doctors were based on what they learned in this training. Now, however, the ideal practice is based on information that has been tested scientifically through experiments and trials. At issue is the validity of the experiments and trials.

In the field of infertility, the best evidence comes from prospective, randomized, placebo-controlled trials. A "prospective" trial means the researcher asks questions such as: Will the drug being evaluated increase fertility? Then patients are enrolled in a trial.

Reporting research always has the potential for bias. For example, a particular drug therapy may have been offered to a group that was too small or to a group that did not include a sufficiently broad spectrum of medical issues. Ultimately, reporting on such experiences can either overestimate or underestimate success potential. The message is that there are no easy answers to complex issues.

So, for example, how do you ascertain whether information on the Internet or in a book is correct? First, look for additional information that confirms what you have found. If there seems to be a general medical consensus, there is a far better chance the information is accurate.

Second, consider the source of the information. If it quotes from articles published in respected journals such as *Fertility & Sterility* or *Human Reproduction*, there is a much better chance of legitimacy. At the very least, you can look up the source and analyze the data yourself. If, on the other hand, supporting data are not available, whatever you have found may not be accurate.

Third, consider the motives of the source – particularly websites. Are you satisfied the data were subjected to the scrutiny of "peer review" whereby other professionals with no financial motive reviewed it? The professional journals just cited (and others as well) require a rigorous peer-review process before an article is published.

A couple of other points are important as well: Look for websites that are all about information. They have no commercial ax to grind. Think carefully about any site that is really trying to sell you something under the guise of providing information. The Centers for Disease Control and Prevention website (www.cdc.gov) and infertility advocacy group website (www.resolve.com) are examples of noncommercial sites that serve the public with good information.

Finally, the professional credential of board certification is one more indicator that information is solid.

Choosing the right doctor for you

This is the most important choice you will make in your quest to overcome infertility. With all due respect to your local phone company, don't make this choice by going to the Yellow Pages.

First, understand that what you're embarking on is both a science and an art. Treating infertility issues involves the science of medicine and the art of strong interpersonal relationships.

The science aspect represents technology-based diagnosis and corrective procedures to make the connection between a sperm and an egg. But because of the intensely personal nature of infertility issues, there is also an art to the connection between patient and doctor as well as patient and nurse.

Creating each of those connections ultimately includes both high-tech and high-touch. You'll want to find an infertility practice that excels at both.

You'll also want to find one with excellent credentials. Medicine – particularly in complex areas such as infertility – involves issues that require judgment and skills that can be learned only over time.

In addition to experience, look for a busy practice. Generally speaking, it is to your advantage to be one of a substantial volume of patients with similar problems. You want to be certain the infertility doctor you are considering is part of a practice that can address a full array of both female and male factor infertility issues with all of the potential solutions, including in vitro and perhaps donor and surrogacy programs.

The last thing you want to do with respect to anything as challenging and stressful as infertility is to have to change doctors because you originally selected a practice without checking it out carefully.

The importance of "board-certified"

The official board certification for infertility is in reproductive endocrinology. This is because most specialists treat women with reproductive disorders even 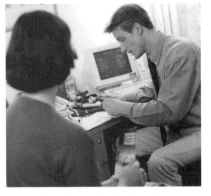 if they are not presently seeking infertility treatment. For example, a woman who has polycystic ovary syndrome – a condition that causes irregular periods and perhaps hirsutism (excessive facial or body hair) – may consult a reproductive endocrinologist even though the problem for which she's seeking help isn't a fertility issue.

The ASRM website has a section labeled Society for Reproductive Endocrinology and Infertility, which lists board-certified infertility specialists. The website also spells out the details of board certification. This designation is your best assurance that a doctor you are considering is both experienced and respected.

"Board-certified" means an independent group of medical specialists has evaluated an individual physician. At the time this book was being written, ASRM noted that "fewer than 800 physicians have achieved this very special distinction." Generally, certification is for a specified period, after which a doctor must be recertified.

In the case of infertility, a board-certified specialist is certified in general obstetrics and gynecology in addition to infertility. This implies that the doctor has successfully completed specialized training in infertility and reproductive endocrinology. If you conclude from this that some physicians may be board-certified in obstetrics and gynecology but not infertility – and that they still manage infertility patients – you are correct. You need to decide whether that is appropriate for your situation.

Most people with infertility issues start with their OB/GYN for initial counseling, investigation, and some level of treatment. If they are not successful, many will subsequently seek out an infertility specialist.

Once you have made your choice and consulted with an infertility specialist, ask some questions about the structure of the program before proceeding:

- **How many specialists are in the group?**

- **Which one will be my principal doctor?**

- **What is the role of the nurses?**

- **Whom should I call with a question?**

Finally, when you choose an infertility specialist, you really choose an entire support team. At the very least, this team includes physician specialists, nurses, an ultrasound technologist, psychologists, laboratory personnel, and a financial counselor. Again, this points to the importance of selecting a practice with enough breadth and depth to address all of your needs.

In particular, be sure that your physician team includes a urologist who is experienced with male infertility issues.

With respect to the laboratory personnel, make certain they include an embryologist (who is involved in techniques to obtain an embryo) and an andrologist (who analyzes and prepares sperm for in vitro fertilization or for insemination). Often, a laboratory director is trained in both of these specialized areas.

And the psychologists should have a broad view of managing the many stresses associated with infertility treatment.

One more thing: Once you have a treatment plan, you may have some doubts. If that is the case, don't hesitate to get a second opinion. What you are doing is far too important to allow doubts to linger.

Checking on outcomes

Information on patient outcomes is available on the Internet as provided by the Centers for Disease Control and Prevention. The CDC posts this cautionary statement with its data: "A comparison of clinic success rates may not be meaningful because patient medical characteristics and treatment approaches vary from clinic to clinic." The disclaimer is there because you cannot directly compare one place with another. The populations are very different. However, it is always worthwhile to see the results of a center. So if it claims a higher pregnancy rate, the patient can ask why the official report says differently. We would also add that the CDC postings are for infertility centers, not individual doctors. When you go to www.cdc.gov, click on ART Success Rates to look into the issue of outcomes.

A few words about cost

The financial costs associated with infertility issues are significant, so much so that we have devoted an entire chapter to that topic. Please see Chapter 10.

For now, suffice it to say this can be a real issue for anyone who does not have insurance coverage for such procedures. Unfortunately, nearly everyone falls into that category. Most people are not covered.

That leads to the delicate subject of "bargain hunting." There is always somebody somewhere who will do something at a lower cost. Probably a good rule of thumb is to avoid the temptation to shop price. You want to give yourself the best chance for success. That means you want to become a patient of a very good infertility practice.

Get a referral

Some of our patients are self-referrals, but most are referred to us by either their gynecologist or their family doctor.

Ask for a referral to a good infertility specialist in your area. Your doctor knows you ultimately will be coming back. That doctor will want you to have the best possible experience.

Friends are another source of referrals. Perhaps you have friends with infertility issues who are willing to share their experiences with a nearby infertility practice. That is worth your attention.

- **•Ask your friends about the quality of patient-doctor communications.**

- **•Ask whether they believe their case was handled thoughtfully throughout.**

- **•Ask whether they would recommend you go to that doctor.**

But don't ask them technical medical questions they are not qualified to answer. Save those for the doctor.

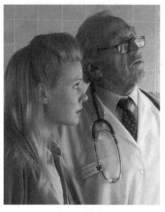

Good chemistry

Ultimately, the relationship between patient and doctor (really, between patient and the full medical staff) must feel right. There should be a comfort factor. The relationship must "fit."

As with most relationships, that fit is often based on good communication. If the communication is lacking, the relationship will not be as productive as you want it to be. Early on, make sure the communication is good, especially with respect to the highly trained nurses who will be your day-to-day link.

Good communication is not a one-way street. You have just as much responsibility to be candid and open as do the doctor and staff. Say what is on your mind. Ask what you want to know about. Demand the same from them.

Summary

There is a great deal of information out there. Some of that information is very good; some of it is not so good. It's essential to know the difference.

Be especially skeptical of information on websites that are not sponsored by professional societies, the government, or respected patient advocacy groups.

Depend on your friends for information about their experiences with doctors, but do not ask them medical questions they have not been trained to answer. Get the medical information you need from medical people.

Likewise, there are many doctors who will be happy to treat you. Some of those doctors are extremely well qualified to do that. Some are not. Do the homework so that you end up in the right hands. Do all you can to work with a board-certified physician. Never forget that a good infertility practice is more than one doctor. It is an entire team that knows how to address all of the complex issues associated with infertility.

Once you select your doctor, it is time to find out what you need to do to achieve your goal – a baby. The next several chapters address that in some detail.

Chapter 3

Preventing Infertility from Happening to You

*"Results are what you expect;
consequences are what you get."*
— Anonymous

That is an appropriate quote to begin this important chapter. It is worth restating that quote in the context of infertility: If you want good treatment results, understand that there are consequences to the way you behave along the way.

You might ask why anybody who wants to be a parent would do anything to put that goal at risk. That is a reasonable question. Yet people do just that every day. And we see people like that all the time in our practice.

So if "today is the first day of the rest of your life," then today is a very good day to get focused on doing everything you can to prevent infertility from happening to you. That's EVERYTHING in capital letters. There are many ways you can improve your chances for the outcome you want.

When people talk about infertility, the focus is almost always on getting pregnant. Yes, that is goal one. It is the first step and it is the subject of this book.

But your focus needs to be much broader than that. What you are seeking to do is about far more than just conceiving. It is about four critically important goals:

Goal One: Become pregnant.

Goal Two: Maintain a successful pregnancy to full term.

Goal Three: Do all you can to have the easiest possible delivery.

Goal Four: Give birth to a healthy baby.

That's the program. And in many respects, it is a self-help program. Your lifestyle needs to be consistent with your goals.

Any experienced specialist in our field will tell you that infertility is an issue where you have little or no control in a traditional sense. You cannot force an egg and a sperm to unite. You cannot make an embryo implant in a uterus. You cannot absolutely control those things.

But maximizing your potential to prevent infertility in the first place, achieve pregnancy, have a good pregnancy and delivery, and give birth to a healthy baby are all issues in which you – as an individual – can have significant control. This does not mean you will succeed. But it does mean you are giving yourself – and your baby – the best possible chance.

Plain talk

Nurse-midwife Char Frires tells this story:

"I had a phone call from a woman in our program. She had just finished a round of drug therapy we had prescribed and was getting ready to move on to a super ovulation attempt.

"The woman told me that she and some friends were going to go out after work that day and drink some margaritas. She was calling me because one of her friends had told her she shouldn't be doing that. The woman thought her friend was kidding and that she didn't see any reason why she couldn't even have two margaritas if that's what she felt like doing. She wanted to know what I thought.

"I told her that alcohol, smoking, lack of exercise, and a negative attitude all decrease your chances to conceive. She challenged that. She was furious. I told her she should be maximizing her potential, but that it was up to her which path she chose.

"Finally, I said, 'Go ahead and have a margarita. Then put off your super ov cycle another three months and get yourself back in shape. Take vitamins. Eat real food. Quit smoking.' She hung up on me.

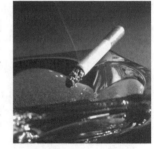

"She called back later and asked if I was really serious about all this. I said, 'Let's change places. You sit at my desk. I'll sit in your chair. What are you going to tell me?'

"My patient said, 'I'll tell you not to smoke and drink and to exercise if you want to have a healthy baby.'"

Point made?

Medically speaking

Prevention of infertility problems is the first objective. It is important that men and women have the facts about the causes of infertility and then make an informed decision about how they want to proceed.

Individual behavior has an absolute impact on the four most common causes of infertility:

- Infertility risks associated with sexually transmitted diseases.

- Infertility risks associated with excessive or too little body weight.

- Infertility risks associated with alcohol and smoking.

- Infertility risks associated with advancing age of the woman.

Not only are these problems frequently the root cause of infertility, they may well be associated with poorer results from infertility treatments. For example, if a woman with a sexually transmitted disease has infertility from blocked uterine tubes, the presence of a severely dilated tube (hydrosalpinx) can decrease the success of in vitro fertilization. This condition can result from an STD. It is a fact that STDs are by far the most common cause of infertility.

STDs and infertility

The most frequently associated STDs seen with infertility patients are chlamydia and gonorrhea.

Just in the United States, 12 million cases of STDs are acquired each year with three-quarters occurring in patients after their teenage years. These bacteria are acquired exclusively through unprotected sexual intercourse and are preventable by adopting safe sexual patterns – especially the use of condoms.

Infection of the uterine tubes is called pelvic inflammatory disease (PID). After one episode of PID, an estimated 13 percent of women become infertile. After three episodes of PID, 75 percent of women become infertile. The most common cause of PID is a sexually transmitted disease, specifically chlamydia or gonorrhea. There are an estimated 3 million new cases of chlamydia in the United States each year.

Unfortunately, most episodes of PID are termed "subclinical." What that means is that most patients do not seek treatment because the symptoms are mild – tolerable lower abdominal pain or a moderately more painful period. The disease becomes self-limiting and the symptoms subside. If high blood pressure can be referred to as a "silent killer," these STDs can be silent obstacles – as in obstacles that prevent you from getting pregnant.

There are indeed consequences associated with our behavior.

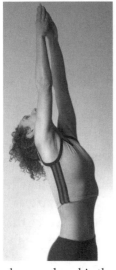

Body weight and proper nutrition

Extremes of body weight – too much or too little – are often associated with infertility as well as poorer outcomes from infertility treatment.

A person's weight is related to a person's height. The parameter used to describe this relationship is called the body mass index or BMI. For those of you with a technical bent, BMI is the weight in kilograms divided by the height in meters squared. It also can be calculated this way: Multiply your weight in pounds by 703. Divide your answer by your height in inches. Again, divide your answer by your height in inches. The number you get is your BMI. Any BMI under 18.5 or over 24.9 is considered abnormal and is therefore potentially problematic for your ability to conceive.

In clinical practice, excess body weight is the most frequent problem, but we also see a substantial population of underweight women. Eating disorders associated with severely underweight women can be extremely dangerous. These patients have many medical problems. One is disruption of the menstrual cycle, which leads to lack of ovulation. Even attempting pregnancy in a severely underweight woman can be dangerous to both the mother and baby. To achieve normal body weight, treatment requires both a medical specialist and a counselor. With treatment in place, the menstrual period will usually normalize. However, if that does not happen, medication may help induce ovulation after ideal body weight is achieved.

Today, 60 percent of American adults are either overweight (BMI 25-29) or obese (BMI over 30). There are websites you can access to calculate your BMI index. Two are www.nhlbisupport.com/bmi and www.nhlbi.nih.gov/guidelines/obesity/bmi_tbl.htm.

It is a fact that excess body weight is related to excess calories. However, a study comparing Italian women with American women found a higher weight in American women despite similar caloric intake. The difference was attributed to lifestyle factors such as the more sedentary habits of American society. This clearly underscores the importance of exercise in maintaining a good body weight. It is important to get both the body and mind into proper shape to optimize either spontaneous or infertility treatment pregnancy rates. Excess body weight is especially a problem in patients with polycystic ovary syndrome, an endocrine disorder that causes ovulation problems that have a negative impact on fertility potential.

Patients who are obese should have treatment not only for fertility reasons but also for the increased health risks during pregnancy and long-term. Counseling, diet, and exercise are the most important intervention modalities for obese patients.

I don't recommend going on any special diets such as carbohydrate-free diets. The imperative is calorie control. Exercise at least thirty minutes per day, but increase that to sixty to ninety minutes if weight loss is your goal.

The typical recommended serving size is far less than my Italian mother could ever have imagined. Today, a serving of cooked pasta is one-half cup. A typical serving for me when I was growing up was closer to eight cups! So times have changed and a reassessment may be necessary in your case, too.

Dietary guidelines are available online at www.healthierus.gov/dietaryguidelines/. Essentially, these guidelines recommend cutting calories, including exercise in your regular routine, and choosing quality foods.

Whole grains are preferred. Two cups of fruit and two and a half cups of vegetables per day are recommended. Three cups per day of fat-free milk or its equivalent will provide the necessary minerals. Focus on a diet low in both saturated fat and cholesterol. Reduce salt (less than one level teaspoonful per day) and consume less added sugar.

Fish and shellfish may contain high levels of mercury, which comes from industrial pollution and is harmful to an unborn baby. It accumulates in the body and takes a long time to eliminate. Therefore, women trying to conceive should be vigilant in avoiding food that contains mercury. The larger fish – swordfish, shark, king mackerel, and tilefish – have the highest concentration of mercury and should be eliminated from your diet.

But don't completely avoid fish because it's an important food. Two meals per week of canned light tuna, salmon, or pollock are fine. Check these websites for details: www.cfsan.fda.gov or www.epa.gov/ost/fish.

All patients attempting pregnancy should be taking a prenatal supplement that gives the right amounts of vitamins and minerals. In particular, it is essential to be taking adequate amounts of folic acid to help prevent neural tube defects (spinal cord problems). The typical dosage range suggested is 0.4 mg or 400 micrograms. Higher doses may be required in some patients. Vegetarians should also add 3 micrograms of vitamin B12 two or three times each week.

The role of other nutritional supplements, "natural" products, or homeopathic supplements to help fertility is unknown. Most of these products have not been tested in rigorous clinical trials to determine their effectiveness. Evidence that they work is most often anecdotal through patient testimonials, not proper scientific clinical trials. Rather than publication in peer-reviewed journals, articles often simply reflect an author's personal experience. These products are frequently recommended as "supplements" rather than "treatments." This is because drug treatments need approval from the Food and Drug Administration.

What we do know for certain is that such products can have an adverse effect. For example, St. John's Wort can exacerbate the sedative effect of certain drugs. Ginkgo biloba can exacerbate the effect of anticoagulants (commonly referred to as blood thinners). The effectiveness of these supplements has not been studied adequately and they may actually make an existing infertility problem worse.

My recommendation would be to discontinue them if you are on them now and to avoid them altogether if you are not. Either way, let your doctor know.

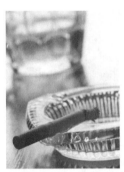

Smoking and alcohol

Smoking is associated with decreased fertility in women. That said, one of my patients told me: "My neighbor smokes a pack of cigarettes per day and has four children."

Clearly, smoking is not by itself a cause of infertility. But neither should it be considered a contraceptive device!

However, smoking is associated with lower fertility rates and has been shown in every study to decrease the desired results of infertility treatment. This is at times quite dramatic as with in vitro fertilization.

Smoking accelerates the natural loss of eggs (oocytes). Even secondhand smoke has been shown to negatively affect fertility and to decrease fertility treatment success rates. Smoking has been associated with increased miscarriage rates and difficulties with pregnancy. Therefore, your home and if possible your work environment should be smoke-free.

If you are a smoker and you want to address your infertility, start right now with a smoking cessation program. Typically, two months smoke-free is the goal before you start infertility treatment.

Alcohol also has been shown to have a toxic effect on fertility potential. It is difficult to know whether there is a lower consumption limit where there is no effect on pregnancy rates. The same general concept applies to caffeine. To be on the safe side, we recommend that all alcohol and caffeine be avoided. At the risk of stating the obvious, this prohibition also extends to recreational drugs.

Reproductive aging

As discussed in the first chapter – and worthy of more in-depth discussion here as well as throughout this book – there is a natural decrease in fertility with a woman's advancing age. The older you are, the less your pregnancy potential.

Women are most fertile in their 20s and 30s.

Women under the age of 25 years have a pregnancy rate at six months of 60 percent and at one year of 85 percent. Compare that to women 35 years or older who will take twice as long to reach the same percentages (60 percent probability of pregnancy at one year and 85 percent at two years).

The decline is not linear and accelerates after the age of 37. Spontaneous pregnancies or pregnancies with infertility treatment are markedly decreased after the age of 40.

This decline relates to the biological fact that women are born with a fixed number of eggs. Those eggs are depleted at the time of menopause. The peak number of eggs is found in the ovary of a fetus. By birth those eggs have decreased to one to two million and by puberty there are only 300,000 eggs left. This loss accelerates further after age 37 even if ovulation is prevented, such as with use of the birth-control pill.

But it is not just about the quantity of a woman's eggs. The quality of the remaining eggs also diminishes over time. The eggs associated with the most fertile potential are depleted first so that with increasing age, the follicle pool is also less fertile.

The impact of egg quality is seen in the embryos derived from them. An abnormal chromosome number (referred to as aneuploidy) is seen in half the embryos that look completely normal under the microscope. In other words, it is "normal" for a woman over 40 to have a large number of "abnormal" embryos. That is not a good thing.

Factors such as smoking, ovarian surgery, or some types of drugs such as those associated with chemotherapy treatment may accelerate this egg-aging process.

A woman's uterus does not seem to "age" to the same degree since embryos that come from eggs of a younger woman can be transferred into an older woman with the same fertility success rates as for younger women.

That is balanced by the fact that miscarriages increase with age. At least 40 percent of women over the age of 40 who do achieve pregnancy will have a miscarriage. This high number compares with a 10 percent miscarriage rate for women younger than 30.

As women grow older, there is also a greater chance of developing other disorders such as endometriosis or fibroids (myomas) that may also contribute to an infertility problem.

Environmental pollutants

Environmental pollutants such as dioxins and pesticides have been shown in animal studies to be associated with infertility or diseases that cause infertility. Dioxins are byproducts of industrial processing. Patients are exposed through their diet. Such contaminants are called hormone disruptors. These agents bind to hormone receptors and disrupt their signals. There may even be a permanent alteration of genes important in child development. Dioxins have been shown to cause endometriosis in animal models.

There is biological plausibility as to why these pollutants can cause endometriosis in humans. However, extrapolating these findings to humans is more problematic. Today, environmental pollution is so prevalent that it would be difficult to find a population not exposed at some level. That makes it very difficult to evaluate the contribution of pollution to infertility.

We believe that most of the causes of infertility are related directly to the causes discussed earlier and that pollutants are not commonly the single cause of an infertility problem. They don't help, but they are not the principal villain.

Infertility and stress

Stress – both mental and physical – has always been associated with infertility. It has long been recognized that infertility and especially its treatment may lead to anxiety and depression. However, only recently has mental stress been shown to have an impact on infertility treatment outcome and actually contribute to the infertility problem.

Physical stress such as that associated with illness will affect reproductive organs. For example, patients with active Crohn's disease, an inflammatory bowel dis-

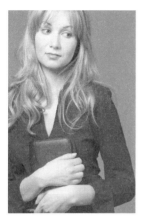

order, can have disruption of the mechanisms in the brain that control ovaries or testes. Women with Crohn's disease often will not ovulate properly and will notice abnormalities in their menstrual cycle – especially the length of time from one menstrual flow to the next. Although men will not notice much on the surface, sperm production will be greatly affected. Furthermore, because sperm produced is ejaculated two or three months later, a semen analysis may not show the abnormal counts until after the man has already recovered from an illness.

It is hard to determine what comes first with regard to the stress associated with infertility. A woman has tremendous stress in her life when conception is not happening. The stress frequently carries over to her partner and can affect their sex life and overall relationship. Sex on a schedule decided by an ovulation kit is not the most romantic way to create a child. The anxiety of the man having sex on demand can definitely be stressful to the couple.

Stress also comes inadvertently from family and friends inquiring about when the couple is going to have children. This is most difficult at events such as baby showers or a birthday party for another couple's child.

Stress can result from a perception that the problem is the fault of one member of the couple only. Most often, that is simply not true. In addition, the financial commitments associated with infertility treatment often cause tremendous stress for couples as do actions that go contrary to ethical or religious beliefs.

Stress can even originate from an employer who may not understand or appreciate the strict time requirements of infertility treatment. Even if you are inclined to be a private person, you may find it extremely difficult to keep your infertility confidential in the workplace if you are regularly going in for tests or treatments.

It is entirely clear to medical professionals that stress does occur in all couples when infertility is present. We also know that stress can negatively affect fertility outcomes.

Other than the typical stress-related symptoms such as anxiety and depression, hostility may be exhibited by you or your stressed-out partner. Headaches, insomnia, and fatigue are other symptoms. We know that depressive disorders may occur as well. Therefore, it is vitally important to recognize these problems and get support. That support can come from many sources, including family, friends, and infertility support groups.

The next level is to work with a therapist for stress management. A good rule of thumb is: Don't fight counseling. Get it if you need it.

Those patients who seek counseling are taught relaxation exercises and coping skills. Acupuncture is effective for some patients. There are also centers referred to as "mind/body" infertility programs that offer these services. They are often very effective.

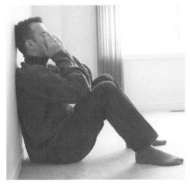

Male factor infertility

No specific cause is found in 30 to 50 percent of male infertility. Smoking, body weight, and age do not have as much of an impact on male infertility as on female infertility. However, it is generally accepted that these factors have enough of an impact that lifestyle modification such as weight loss and smoking cessation is warranted. Smoking is the most critical of these factors because of the effect of secondhand smoking on female fertility potential.

With advanced paternal age, there may be some small increase in chromosomal problems in the embryo. Men between the ages of 45 and 69 have lower semen parameters than younger men, but they are always in the normal range. On the other hand, male factor infertility often has a significant genetic component.

Pre-evaluation tests and recommendations

Before consulting with an infertility specialist and even before attempting pregnancy, a woman should be evaluated by her primary-care provider. During this visit, she should discuss the medications she's on; some may have to be changed or stopped altogether. Some "natural" products may have to be stopped, too, as these can actually decrease fertility. Most lubricants are spermicidal and should not be used.

On the other hand, an antenatal vitamin that includes folic acid should be started.

Here are other steps to take:

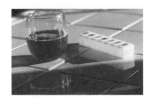

- Breast and pelvic exams as well as a Pap test should be up to date.

- Make sure immunizations are current.

- Be certain you are rubella-immune since exposure to this infection can cause congenital birth defects. In addition to the rubella titer, basic tests that should be considered include blood type and antibody screen. HIV and hepatitis B screen also should be considered.

- See your dentist for a checkup and cleaning.

Some genetic tests should be considered as well. These tests are often specific to ethnic groups, such as screening for sickle-cell anemia for African Americans; Tay-Sachs and Canavan Disease for Ashkenazi Jews; beta thalassemia (blood disorder) for people of southern Mediterranean descent (such as Greek or Italian); alpha thalassemia (blood disorder) for Asians (such as Chinese); and cystic fibrosis for all patients. These tests are often done at a first prenatal visit. In the context of infertility treatment, it is always advantageous to know about such issues up front.

The children of patients who are of Irish descent may have an increased risk of neural tube defects, which is a disorder of the spinal cord. However, there is no specific blood test before pregnancy to investigate this. The test for neural tube defects is done during pregnancy. That limitation aside, your physician may recommend a higher dose of folic acid, typically 4 mg, to address this potential issue as early as possible in a preventive mode.

The rate of spontaneous congenital anomalies in newborns is between 2 and 4 percent. The risk of chromosomally abnormal children increases with increasing age of the woman. Although increasing age of the man may also carry this risk, it is far smaller. The couple should consult with their obstetrician about appropriate options for antenatal diagnosis of chromosomal problems such as amniocentesis or chorionic villus sampling.

This is also the optimal time to find out whether there are genetic problems in the family. Either person can be a carrier. For example:

- Is there any family history of mental retardation? A syndrome, called Fragile X, could be the cause.

- Are there family members with birth defects such as those of the spine?

- Are there an unusual number of cancers?

It is important to discuss these types of issues with your obstetrician before consulting an infertility specialist so that they can be evaluated to the extent possible in advance of pregnancy. Of course, the infertility doctor is trained to investigate these problems as well, but that will only delay the initiation of infertility treatment if you wait until then.

If either partner has a medical problem, such as high blood pressure, it is also recommended that a consultation occur with the physician responsible for managing this disorder to ensure that the condition is optimized and all medication reviewed for potential harmful effects to the fetus. This is especially the case in a woman with some of these problems. Clearly, she needs to know the risk of carrying a pregnancy.

Finally, a mammogram is recommended once between the age of 35 and 40, then yearly after the age of 40. Starting earlier than 35 may be necessary for women with a higher risk of breast cancer. Check with your doctor on this before you start infertility treatment.

Front-line perspectives

Doctors, nurses, counselors, allied health-care professionals, and a variety of support personnel get very close to our patients. In fact, they are often the front-line troops. Throughout this book, we will feature their perspectives. Here, for example, are some thoughts from one of our physicians.

Although this chapter and, indeed, this book are basically about getting you pregnant, you need to be looking beyond that to also start – right now – maximizing your potential to produce a healthy baby once you become pregnant.

If the first goal is to get you pregnant, it is also appropriate at this point to focus briefly on your three other goals: maintaining a successful pregnancy, having the easiest possible delivery, and giving birth to a healthy baby.

Elliot Philipson, M.D., is a maternal-fetal medicine specialist. He leads our subspecialty group that manages high-risk pregnancies and obstetric complications. What he has to say merits your attention both now and later.

"The infertility staff gets them pregnant. Then, it's our job to get those tough cases through pregnancy and, hopefully, to deliver a healthy baby or babies.

"If you want to help yourself and your baby, key issues are to avoid drinking and smoking, watch your weight, eat right, and exercise.

"One of the things we try to do is to help women be nutritionally sound and stable by eating a healthy diet and using both a good multivitamin and folic acid. There are a lot of health-food crazes and alternative diets out there. We don't have studies that indicate how those impact a pregnancy. So avoid them. Eat a regular balanced diet and take the vitamin supplements your doctor recommends.

"Why do we worry so much about these types of issues? Well, here are two good examples.

"One is that we know that diabetes in the mom increases the risk of congenital malformation of the baby. Glucose or sugar control is the cornerstone of diabetes management. Your weight and watching what you eat are important

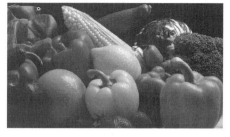

to addressing that.

"Secondly, we know that smoking can result in smaller babies as the nicotine can constrict the small blood vessels and decrease blood flow to the fetus. So we worry a lot about smoking and even secondary smoke. Those are just two examples of how lifestyle can impact a pregnancy.

"Using the proper medications in the right amounts is another big issue. If, for example, somebody has chronic hypertension, we would want the patient to have normal blood pressure and have that issue under control during a pregnancy. So we might recommend changing some of the medications to get that to happen. Another example might be a woman who suffers from migraine headaches and who might be taking something that can be harmful during a pregnancy. We might change that, too.

"Something you want to be especially careful of during a pregnancy is what we call 'self-medicating,' which is when patients make changes in drug therapy without consulting a physician. That can be very, very harmful. Sometimes women who are affected by chronic depression will stop taking medication on their own because of something they read on the Internet. Don't do that. Always ask your doctor what you should or should not be taking. Even for a simple headache, know that you should take acetaminophen and you should not take conventional aspirin if you are pregnant.

"Lots of people who come to me have very high stress levels – particularly if they have been in an infertility program for a long time.

"Large population studies show that as a woman gets older, the chances of having a baby with Down syndrome or other chromosomal abnormalities increase. It is not a straight-line curve. The older the mom gets after that, the higher the risk. For example, at age 35, it might be 1 in 270 pregnancies, but as you get into your 40s, that risk can increase to 1 in 20, or 5 percent of pregnancies. Compare those statistics with age 30 when the risk is only 1 in 1,000.

"It's important to understand these complex issues. One of the questions you should be asking your OB/GYN is this: 'Does my racial or ethnic background indicate I have any special risks?' For example, there is a higher risk of giving birth to a baby with cystic fibrosis if you are of northern European descent. Learn all you can about these risks. Ask questions. Get answers."

Frequently asked questions

We subscribe to the belief that "there are no dumb questions." Every question deserves a thoughtful response geared to the individual situation of the person asking it, and answers might vary depending on the individual situation.

The following are questions we hear from many patients. You may want to ask them of your own doctor.

Q. Is there a risk that somebody can get obsessed with all the healthy lifestyle advice to the point where that becomes unhealthy?

A. It will be unhealthy only if the stress of "perfection" leads to anxiety.

Q. Should I crank up my exercise program if I want to get pregnant, or should I lower it or just basically leave it the same?

A. A healthy lifestyle implies regular exercise, and that should be initiated immediately. (Follow the guidelines discussed earlier in this chapter.)

Q. With respect to exercise, are there any special risks for infertility patients versus people who don't have that issue?

A. For in vitro fertilization patients, it may be prudent to refrain from intense exercise during the time of the largest increase in ovarian size. However, walking is always fine.

Q. What should I absolutely quit doing if I want to get pregnant?

A. We look at smoking as the number one predator. Some infertility programs will not accept women in an in vitro fertilization program until they have quit smoking.

Q. If I quit smoking, I might put on weight. Is quitting smoking a good trade-off for increased weight?

A. Stop smoking first. Keep weight off by exchanging cigarettes for exercise. We can deal with weight problems better than we can with cigarette problems.

Q. Is it okay to be a vegetarian if I want to get pregnant, or should I force myself to eat meat?

A. Being a vegetarian is fine. Just be sure to eat legumes, such as beans, that are high in protein. And take a vitamin supplement.

Q. What are some simple steps you recommend that can reduce stress, including my stress about infertility?

A. Recognize that you and your partner are a team. Don't blame each other or yourself for the infertility problem. Avoid activities that cause increased stress, such as going to a baby shower. Maintain other interests you had before and continue to enjoy the things you enjoyed before coming to see us.

Q. Isn't it basically true that everything done or taken in moderation is probably okay?

A. There is no "moderation" when it comes to cigarettes or other unhealthy habits.

Patient talk

We believe that one of the greatest services this book can provide is to connect readers with the actual experiences of Cleveland Clinic patients. For reasons of patient confidentiality, we have changed their names. But the experiences are real. Look for these case histories in several chapters. Here is the first one.

Like all couples with infertility challenges, Allie and Bob experienced "the agony of defeat" many times before experiencing "the thrill of victory." This is what they went through.

"After all the tests, we fell into the category called 'unexplained infertility.' In our case, the diagnosis was that there is no precise diagnosis. As you can imagine, that can be very frustrating.

"Our case was further complicated by the fact that my husband had inherited several genetic disorders that had nothing to do with fertility – except that they could become an issue if I were to ultimately give birth. A genetic counselor explained which disorders were 'dominant' and 'recessive' and presented us with statistics. It was clearly better not to pass those issues on to the next generation.

"To address his genetic issues, everyone agreed the only safe course was to use donor sperm. Care was taken to identify a prospective donor matching physical and ethnic characteristics with my husband as closely as possible.

"For me to have the best chance to become pregnant, I was put on injectable drug therapy to enhance prospects for good eggs and successful ovulation. The first drug caused some burning at the injection site. A second drug had no noticeable side effects and led to the desired result.

"Over time, my legs became swollen and sore from the injections. I experienced mood swings from all the hormones. It is so easy to become depressed when those things happen. However, I always believed in my heart of hearts that eventually we would have success. I was able to persevere with the ongoing support of my husband and medical team.

"Did we have concerns? Yes. There were many fears related to the unknown. My infertility drugs had only been on the market a very short time (mid-1990s). There was no data available yet to show long-term side effects. We were concerned about potential birth defects. I was 38 years old, the odds of having a healthy baby were declining, and taking fertility drugs was worrisome. We also worried about the donor sperm process, including whether the donor had been truthful with all the information on his application.

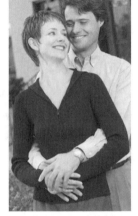

"But after confronting those issues and after much careful thought, we chose not to share the information about the donor sperm or infertility treatment with our extended family. We're very glad we made that decision. We went forward with donor sperm and IUI (intrauterine insemination). At the age of 39, I gave birth to our first child.

"We decided to try again two years later. I was now 41. What worked in my earlier pregnancy did not work this time. After using super ovulation, I did not have any usable eggs even for in vitro. I was advised not to undergo further drug therapy. It was too late. The odds of success were less than 1 percent.

"Following that prognosis, I was asked, 'Have you considered adoption?'

"Today, we have two active, healthy children. Our older child was conceived through super ovulation and IUI using donor sperm. Our younger child was adopted from overseas.

"The stress of not getting pregnant is very tough. It's dreadful when you want a family and you're almost 40, all of your friends have children, and you begin to believe you may never experience that. Really, nobody can truly understand what you're going through unless they've been there. But there was just something inside of me that said, 'Don't be afraid. Keep going. This is where you're supposed to go.'"

Summary

You can, should, and must take steps to help prevent infertility. Put another way, do all you can to maximize your own fertility potential.

The four most frequent causes of infertility are STDs, weight/nutrition, alcohol and smoking, and the age of the woman. You can have a significant impact on those.

Stress is another big issue. Run toward counseling, not away from it.

Finally, understand that getting pregnant is only goal one. You need to stay pregnant, give birth, and bring a healthy child into the world. All of those goals are affected by lifestyle choices.

Please make smart choices.

Chapter 4

Finding the Problem
(Investigation of the Infertile Couple)

> *"Enthusiasm for one's goal lessens the disagreeableness of working toward it."*
> – Thomas Eakins

We are often asked whether the process of diagnosing the infertile couple starts with the woman or the man.

Without being facetious, the answer is yes.

We normally go down a dual track at the outset, making our initial evaluations pretty much simultaneously.

In many cases, only the woman has the infertility issue. In many cases, it is just the man. Other times – in fact, frequently – both the woman and the man face these challenges. Even in situations where one partner owns the primary issue, both may still need treatment.

Plain talk

In the case of women, most issues fall into these categories:

- Problems related to ovulation (failure to produce fertile eggs).

- Blockages somewhere in the reproductive system that interfere with an egg and a sperm uniting.

- A variety of diseases and infectious conditions that can interfere with fertility.

There may be other factors, but those are the most common. And it is not unusual for there to be some combination of these issues. Most of the women we see in our practice match up to at least one of these major categories.

Something we know for certain is that men are very often the cause of infertility. This reinforces the need for men to be just as involved as women in solving infertility challenges.

This means more than just supporting one's spouse. It means a real commitment on the part of men to face up to diagnosis and whatever treatment options ultimately may be dictated for them.

Unlike with women, age is not an infertility issue for men. A 38-year-old man is not faced with the same ticking biological clock. The issues are all sperm-related, but not age-based. Are there enough sperm? Sometimes, in fact, there are no sperm at all. Frequently, the man has an extremely low sperm count. This is an important male infertility issue.

Some patients become really upset with this diagnosis because they feel it means they are less than men. Wrong. There are many contributing factors to this common condition. A low sperm count can often be addressed successfully. And even when that is not the case, an abnormally low sperm count is not a sexual performance issue.

Even if there are enough sperm, are they strong enough to get through both the male and female reproductive systems to end up where they need to be? The term that addresses that issue is known as "motility," which basically determines whether the sperm are able to move as they should.

There is another important word that also happens to start with the letter M. That word is "morphology," and it deals with the structure of sperm. A healthy shape is critical to the ability of a tiny sperm to penetrate an egg. So we look at this as well.

Even if the number, strength, and shape of sperm appear satisfactory, there is another set of potential male complications that can lead to infertility.

Is there some condition in the male plumbing system, such as a blockage, disease, or infection, which inhibits the ability of sperm to move along as they should? If so, what is it and what needs to be done about it? Again, this is a very common diagnosis.

Other issues can have an impact on male fertility. These include genetic and environmental factors.

So just as a good detective follows leads, a couple wanting to seriously address infertility must determine whether there is a male factor contributing to their lack of success. That process starts with what is known as a semen analysis.

Our job is to take a thoughtful approach to identifying any issue(s) and to suggest equally thoughtful responses that provide you and your spouse with the most appropriate way to achieve your goal – a baby. Your job is to stay involved, listen carefully, and then actively participate in the decisions that may help you.

With respect to the so-called "developed" countries, the World Health Organization has reported that infertility can be attributed as follows:

- A problem for both partners in 40 percent of the cases.
- A problem exclusive to the woman in 40 percent of the cases.
- A problem exclusive to the man in 10 percent of the cases.
- A problem that cannot be clearly identified ("unexplained infertility") in 10 percent of the cases.

A study done in Canada reported the following distribution:

- A problem exclusive to the woman in 50 percent of the cases.
- A problem exclusive to the man in 24 percent of the cases.
- Unexplained infertility in 26 percent of the cases.

Medically speaking

These results make clear that both women and men should be investigated in the evaluation of infertility. Just because there is an obvious cause of infertility in one partner, that does not preclude investigation of the other.

Basic reproductive physiology

Before consulting a physician, it is recommended that you obtain some basic information about reproductive physiology. There are many good books on this topic.

It will help greatly to grasp the potential causes of infertility if you can understand both the female and male reproductive systems. It will also help if you have at least a basic knowledge of the tests and treatment that may be recommended in your case.

It is important to know that tests and treatments are cycle-specific. This means that they are performed at different times of the menstrual cycle. The menstrual cycle is divided into two phases.

1. The days before ovulation are called "follicular."

2. The days after ovulation are called "luteal."

As you know, a woman's cycle is numbered starting on the first day of the menstrual cycle. So day one is the first day of her full flow. Theoretically then, day fourteen would be the day of ovulation. So a woman with a twenty-eight-day cycle would ovulate on day fourteen, but a woman with a thirty-day cycle would ovulate on day sixteen. The luteal phase can be between ten and sixteen days in length.

For both men and women, their gonads (testicles and ovaries) are controlled by parts of the brain (called hypothalamus and pituitary gland). The pituitary gland secretes follicle-stimulating hormones and luteinizing hormones. These hormones can be measured in the blood.

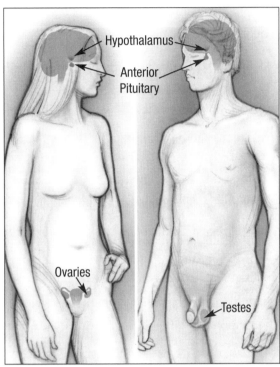

Sorry, but you really do need to become acquainted with a few of these medical terms. Soon they will become second nature. You'll start using them. It is a fact that many patients learn the "medical jargon" so well that they are able to communicate easily with all medical personnel without needing to resort to more conversational terms.

The main hormones secreted from the ovaries are estrogen, progesterone, and inhibin.

Estrogen is secreted throughout the cycle in different concentrations. The main estrogen is called estradiol. This is what is measured in the blood tests you will have.

Progesterone, on the other hand, is secreted only after ovulation. The cells around the eggs secrete these hormones. Once the eggs are depleted – as in menopause – production of these hormones ceases.

Ovulation is triggered by luteinizing hormones (LH). The peak fertility occurs around the periovulatory time. This time is defined as the three to four days around the time LH is released. LH can be measured in blood, saliva, and urine samples.

The main hormones secreted by the testes are testosterone and inhibin. Testosterone is usually secreted normally even if there is no sperm production at all.

With this brief background, it is now time to talk about some action steps.

The initial consultation

The initial consultation with an infertility specialist is action step number one.

Generally speaking, a consultation for infertility should be scheduled if there has been no conception after one year of unprotected intercourse.

Evaluations should occur before one year if there are obvious problems. Here are examples:

- If the woman's menstrual cycle is abnormal with menstruation occurring infrequently or too frequently.

- If there is a history of sexually transmitted disease.

- If the woman has had surgery on the reproductive tract or undergone a treatment that may affect the reproductive tract.

- Women who are over the age of 35 may want to consider an evaluation after six months of attempting pregnancy unsuccessfully.

There are two purposes for the initial consultation:

1. To collect information.

2. To develop an investigation plan.

Central to the information-gathering process will be questions posed to the woman such as these:

- How long have you tried?

- Have you ever been pregnant?

- Do you or your partner have children with each other or a previous partner?

- What type of contraception have you been using?

- What is the frequency of sexual intercourse?

- Are there any problems such as pain associated with intercourse?

- Details about the menstrual cycle are important. For example, at what age did the first period appear? How often does your period come? Is it painful?

- Are there any symptoms that suggest a hormonal problem such as breast secretions that look like milk (galactorrhea), excessive facial or body hair (hirsutism), or acne?

- What is your history with respect to surgeries or medical problems, including STDs?

Similarly, the initial male reproductive evaluation would include questions along these lines:

- Is there any history of undescended testicles (cryptorchidism)?

- Did you experience a childhood illness such as mumps?

- Have you ever had surgery on the testicles or hernia repairs?

- Are there medical problems in your case such as STDs or diabetes?

Both partners should be asked about current medications and their use of over-the-counter, non-prescription drugs.

- Does either partner use tobacco?

- What is the pattern of alcohol consumption?

- Are there any issues with substance abuse?

- Has there been any exposure to environmental toxins such as pesticides that are known to affect fertility?

- Is there a history of genetic disorders on either side?

Typically, this means asking about ancestry and whether there are certain birth defects in the family.

The answers to these questions are one cornerstone to developing a treatment plan. Another cornerstone is a physical exam.

A physical exam is generally performed on the woman. That exam includes both an assessment of weight and any obvious causes of infertility.

Normally, a physical exam for the man is performed only if there is a suspicious reproductive history or an abnormal semen analysis.

The most common causes of female infertility are tubal disease, problems of ovulation, and endometriosis. Cervical problems such as mucus abnormalities or uterine problems such as fibroids occur far less commonly.

As we discuss the tests used to evaluate fertility, it is important to understand the concept of "no predictive value." There are multiple reasons to do a test. The obvious one is to diagnose a problem. The less obvious reason is to assess whether pregnancy will occur spontaneously in spite of this problem. For example, most women with abnormal cervical mucus will achieve pregnancy spontaneously. So assessing this component has little predictive value. In other words, if the test is normal, you can get pregnant and if the test is abnormal most women can still get pregnant spontaneously.

If, however, a test such as the semen analysis tells us that the chance of a spontaneous pregnancy is very small, we then may offer immediate treatment. A test that can give us this information is worthwhile. Finally, there is one other reason we use a test and that is to predict how a patient will respond to treatment.

So when the physician recommends a test, there are some questions you should ask.

- What will this test tell us about the cause of my infertility?

- If the test is abnormal, does this imply that I have a very low chance of getting pregnant on my own?

- Will the result of the test change the management of my case? If you do the test, will you recommend the same treatment whether the test is normal or not normal? For example, if a postcoital test is recommended and the next step is insemination regardless of whether the test is normal, then why do the test?

- What is the point of the test? The tests are often expensive and can be uncomfortable. Certainly, they can be disruptive to a patient's schedule.

- Is this test generally recommended by the fertility medical societies? Organizations such as the American Society for Reproductive Medicine often review evidence and make recommendations as to the value of a particular test.

Infertility tests for women

Hysterosalpingogram

The uterine tubes, or fallopian tubes, are about 10 to 12 cm long (4 to 5 inches) and are attached to the uterus at one end and open inside the abdomen near the ovary. The uterus has two tubes. The fimbriae, or fine extensions at the end of the tubes, pick up the egg from the ovary. These cells have fine, microscopic finger-like projections that line the tubes, which are critical for their proper function. They are damaged by infection.

Fertilization occurs in a part of the tube called the ampulla. The sperm makes it up through the cervix and uterine cavity to meet the egg in the ampulla, which is the part closest to the ovary. The fertilized egg is then transported down the tube into the uterus. The embryo divides as it progresses through the tube. The embryo then enters the uterine cavity for implantation. This process takes days.

As we noted before, the most common cause of tubal disease is an STD – specifically chlamydia or gonorrhea. Tubal infection is frequently referred to as pelvic inflammatory disease because tubal infection often involves other structures around the tube. Additional causes of tubal disease are adhesions from previous surgery such as fibroid removal, ovarian cyst removal, or endometriosis.

Tubal disease can range from mild to severe, depending on how much damage there is to the tube. Typically, we assess whether there is scar tissue (adhesions) and whether the tubal architecture has been maintained. If the disease is severe, the tube can be enlarged and contain fluid. This dilated tube with fluid is called a hydrosalpinx.

The best test to assess the uterine tubes is called a hysterosalpingogram (HSG). This test also assesses the uterine cavity. It is a radiologic (X-ray) assessment that uses an iodine-based radio-opaque contrast. Patients with allergies to iodine should notify their doctor. Since this test does not inject the contrast material intravenously, there is typically no contraindication in iodine-allergic patients. However, with severe iodine allergy, medication can be given before the test to prevent an adverse reaction.

An HSG is performed after a menstrual period, but before ovulation. A regular dose of nonsteroidal anti-inflammatory medication such as ibuprofen 600 mg can be taken one hour before the test to alleviate pain. The test should not be performed if there is an acute infection or if you are potentially pregnant. If there is a possibility that you are pregnant, such as with irregular periods or periods that are abnormal in length or delayed, a pregnancy test should be performed first.

As with all gynecological exams, this test starts by inserting a speculum into the vagina just as when you have your Pap test. The cervix is cleansed. Then dye is injected through the cervix with a small tube. During the injection, the uterus and tubes are visualized with "spot" films. Most infertility doctors perform this test themselves. However, radiologists do perform the procedure in some centers.

The test usually takes five minutes. Patients normally experience a moderate amount of pain, but the pain should quickly go away. Patients can return to work within an hour. If the pain persists or returns later, the doctor should be notified because it may be a sign of infection.

Infection is an uncommon but potential complication. It is especially seen in patients with previous infections of the uterine tubes. There may be some mild bleeding from the procedure. If bleeding becomes heavier, the doctor should be notified. Fever is always abnormal and the doctor should be notified about that as well.

There may be a therapeutic effect of the X-ray. Pregnancy rates seem to go up slightly after this test. No one is sure why this happens, but it may be that fluid from the test flushes out some minor obstruction such as mucus.

If the test is normal, we can accept that there is no tubal disease. This is especially true if there is no history of pelvic infection.

However, some test results may not be accurate. This is especially true if there is blockage of the tubes close to the uterus. This is called a "proximal tubal occlusion." If this is the case, we usually repeat the test in one or two months because spasm of the proximal tube can give a false impression of blockage. If it is still blocked, then an attempt is made radiologically to unblock the tubes.

If the tube is seen and found to be damaged or blocked at the end (distally), the next step is to decide how to treat the problem.

The HSG test also will give a preliminary evaluation of the uterine cavity. Pathology in the cavity of the uterus, such as birth defects or fibroids (myomas), also can be detected.

There are some alternatives to this test. A blood test could measure the antibody to chlamydia. This would tell whether you were exposed to that infection. However, a blood test will not tell you if the tubes are damaged or how severely they may be damaged. Neither will a blood test tell you anything about gonorrhea or other abnormalities of the uterus or tubes.

Sonohysterogram

Another possible approach is to perform a sonohysterogram (SHG) or saline infusion sonohysterogram (SIS). This is an office-based ultrasound procedure that is used to evaluate the uterine cavity more fully. No preparation other than some ibuprofen-like medication is necessary.

This test is performed immediately after a woman's period has ended, but before ovulation. A small catheter is placed in the uterine cavity and water is instilled. A vaginal ultrasound is then performed to view the cavity and walls of the uterus. This test is excellent for determining the presence of fibroids, polyps, or congenital defects of the uterus. The results are immediate and you can return to work right away.

This test is far less painful than the HSG and the patient has no exposure to X-rays. However, it is very difficult to see the tubes, and patency is often inferred by seeing fluid in the abdomen. If you inject water into the uterus and you see it in the abdomen, a tube must be open even though you do not actually see the tube. This test gives no detail of tubal architecture.

Hysteroscopy

This test also can be performed in an office setting and is a direct visualization of the interior of the uterine cavity. Just as with an SHG test, no preparation other than some ibuprofen-like medication is necessary. Likewise, the hysteroscopy test is performed immediately after a period has ended, but before ovulation.

A small camera called a hysteroscope – usually 3 to 4 mm (25 mm equals 1 inch) – is placed through the cervix into the uterine cavity and water is instilled. The cavity is then visualized by looking into the camera or on a monitor that the patient also can see.

This test confirms the results of the SIS so that appropriate intervention can be planned.

A hysteroscopy test can also be used to treat disorders of the uterine cavity such as polyps or fibroids. However, these hysteroscopes are larger in diameter (typically 9 mm) and require some form of anesthesia. Recovery is quite rapid, typically three days. Instruments are used to remove the lesion in the cavity.

Laparoscopy

This is a procedure that is performed in the operating room. A laparoscope is a camera that is inserted into the abdomen. It can be either 5 or 10 mm in diameter. When the laparoscope is in the abdomen, a gas (carbon dioxide) is introduced into the abdomen so that a space is created to see clearly.

Extra incisions of 5 mm are required to insert instruments. These are placed in the lower abdomen. This procedure is generally safe, but there are risks.

A laparoscopy is performed as a diagnostic procedure, but it can also be used to treat a disorder that is seen and is causing the infertility problem. Recovery is usually five to seven days, but when there is extensive disease, it may be longer.

Laparoscopy is an option for patients with no specific cause of their infertility. It is also used to confirm tubal disease that was first seen with an HSG. Repair of the disease also can be accomplished by laparoscopy. In patients with a history of pelvic pain or infection, it also may be used to assess whether there is pelvic disease. The treatment of most diseases that cause infertility can be accomplished by laparoscopy.

Ovarian reserve testing

The decline in fertility with age is attributed to an egg problem. The term ovarian reserve refers to the general concept of the quality and quantity of the remaining eggs. We have a limited ability to evaluate the quality of those eggs. The most widely used test is to measure a blood level for follicle-stimulating hormone (FSH), a hormone produced in the brain by the pituitary gland.

FSH rises as eggs are depleted. This occurs until very high levels of FSH are found in menopausal women (total egg depletion).

FSH stimulates the cells around the ovary to produce estrogen (estradiol) and a hormone called inhibin. As estrogen and inhibin levels go up, they shut off FSH. This is the normal cycle. It is believed that with egg aging, the ability to produce inhibin is compromised and therefore FSH is higher.

Blood tests for FSH and estrogen levels are measured on day three of the cycle. This can be used by itself. Some physicians just use the day-three FSH and estrogen, while others use the more detailed test described next.

Even more information can be obtained if the FSH and estrogen levels are measured again after taking clomiphene citrate 100 mg from day five to nine. The blood test is obtained on day ten. If the day-three or day-ten FSH is above a certain level, a diminished ovarian reserve is diagnosed. If the day-three estradiol is above 80 pg/mL, the day-three FSH may be hard to interpret because the FSH levels may be artificially low. This is because estrogen will reduce FSH. A day-three blood estrogen level that is elevated is associated with a diminished response to treatment. This poor prognosis also is seen even if repeat testing shows a normal value.

Other potential blood tests include measuring inhibin B levels and antimullerian hormone. Currently, these blood tests are not recommended because they are not generally available and there is insufficient information on how to use the results appropriately.

Another potential test for ovarian reserve is the antral follicle count. This test evaluates the presence of small follicles in the ovary by transvaginal ultrasound. A follicle consists of an egg and its surrounding cells. It is from these small antral follicles that one egg will develop in each cycle.

As a woman gets older, there are fewer antral follicles. An ultrasound performed in the early part of the cycle (before day seven) can measure the quantity of these follicles. If there are fewer than five to ten of these follicles, the prognosis for obtaining a pregnancy from infertility treatment decreases.

The next question is: What do we do with all of this information?

It should be used to counsel couples – not to exclude them. With this information, a couple must determine whether the odds of obtaining a pregnancy are too low for the emotional and financial pain that they will have to undergo if they move forward. This is a very important decision point in treating infertility.

Basal body temperature curves

The time-honored way to evaluate ovulation is the basal body temperature test. With this test, the patient takes her temperature orally in the morning, using a special thermometer. She plots this on a chart. Typically, temperature rises with ovulation. This pattern is called biphasic. If the temperature does not rise (monophasic) or the temperature rise in the luteal phase is less than eleven days, this may indicate a problem.

These tests are relatively inexpensive, but are not reliable enough in and of themselves to assess ovulation or any pathology, since many women with abnormal graphs are nevertheless ovulating normally. This is because a temperature rise can occur for reasons other than just ovulation.

Assessment of ovulation with an LH kit

LH is the hormone responsible for ovulation. It is secreted by the pituitary glands and is excreted into the urine. Therefore, it can be measured by using an over-the-counter saliva or urine kit.

According to the kit, the peak fertility for sexual intercourse is from three to four days before the LH kit is positive and up to two days after the kit is positive. These kits should be used to assess the time of peak fertility. Unless they are used to plan inseminations, they do not need to be used in most circumstances. The kits have never been proven to enhance fertility over regular intercourse.

The best correlation with an LH surge is an evening urine test between 4 and 6 p.m. However, the kits are frequently used in the morning.

Serum progesterone

Progesterone is elevated only after ovulation. A blood test for this can be performed in the mid-luteal phase or six to eight days after the LH surge as documented by a urine test.

Ultrasonography

An ultrasound can be performed every few days from day ten of the cycle for the purpose of following a growing follicle. A follicle will grow and then collapse after ovulation. This is easily seen using ultrasound. However, this test requires frequent visits to evaluate the process over time.

Endometrial biopsy

An endometrial biopsy performed in the luteal phase can indicate whether ovulation occurs. However, this test is painful and adds no more information than a simple blood test for progesterone to assess ovulation. It is now known that the test is not sufficiently accurate or reproducible to use routinely for evaluation of an ovulation disorder.

Other tests

There are many other tests that are available but not considered to be relevant for the initial evaluation of infertility. For example, if there is a clear ovulation disorder or specific symptoms, other hormonal tests such as thyroid testing should be done.

A test that is performed infrequently is the post-coital test. This test is performed around ovulation. It was first used in the late 1800s. In this test, cervical mucus is obtained after sexual intercourse and analyzed for the presence of motile sperm. Abnormalities of cervical mucus are rarely the single cause of infertility. Pregnancies occur even when no motile sperm are found in the test. There are no agreed-upon standards of what is normal.

Finally, most modern treatment of infertility includes insemination, which bypasses any cervical problem.

Infertility tests for men

A man is usually assessed by a combination of collecting a reproductive history and two semen analyses one month apart. If normal, no other initial evaluation is required.

The questions for men include the following:

- Is there a history of medical or surgical problems and/or childhood diseases?
- Are you presently using any medication?
- Do you smoke?
- What is your alcohol consumption pattern?
- Is there any pattern of previous drug use?
- What is the genetic history of your family?
- Are you spending too much time in the hot tub?

A history of undescended testicles or surgery on the testicles or groin can point to a male problem as the cause of infertility. Some diseases such as diabetes may cause what we call a retrograde ejaculation. This means that the sperm will go into the bladder rather than come out in the ejaculate.

Difficulties with maintaining an erection or decreased libido can also be associated with male infertility.

Use of anabolic steroids in male athletes can cause infertility.

If it is determined there is an abnormal reproductive history, a full evaluation by a urologist is required.

The semen analysis should be collected by masturbation without use of lubricants. The best sample is one collected onsite near the lab because this eliminates the problems of transport, including the potentially negative effect of temperature change. For a semen analysis, there should be at least two days of abstinence but not more than five to six days before the test.

The initial semen analysis test has several components:

- An assessment of viscosity.
- Acidity (normal pH: 7.2-7.8).
- Semen volume (2-5 mL).
- Motility (50 percent or more).

- Concentration (more than 20 million/mL).

- Total count (more than 40 million).

- Morphology (shape of the sperm).

Sperm shape (morphology) can be assessed two ways. The first is called a Kruger test and assesses the sperm head. If there are more than 14 percent normal sperm, the shape is considered normal. The second is an assessment of the sperm head and tails, which is suggested by the World Health Organization. Normal is over 30 percent.

The trend in this country is to use the Kruger assessment because it can predict subsequent in vitro fertilization success more accurately.

Some infertility centers will automatically also perform an evaluation for white blood cells in the semen. If there are more than 1 million white blood cells (leukocytes), a further evaluation for possible infection or inflammation should be initiated. Other infertility specialists perform this test only if there are clinical signs of infection or inflammation.

The same concept applies to testing for antibodies in the semen. This test should be performed if there is a history of trauma or surgery to the testicles, or if there is abnormal agglutination (sperm coming together in clumps) reported on the semen analysis results.

An abnormal semen analysis does not mean a spontaneous conception cannot occur. However, values indicated outside these ranges do show a trend toward decreased chances of fertility. Obviously, when there is no sperm at all, pregnancy cannot occur.

An abnormal semen analysis should prompt a physical examination and formal evaluation by a urologist to determine causes. For example, cases of testicular cancer may be detected.

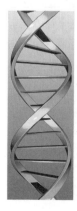

When the concentration is lower than a certain level, a hormonal evaluation should be initiated. These blood tests also can be ordered if there are other suspicious factors in the reproductive history such as impotence. The typical blood tests are follicle-stimulating hormone and testosterone. Other tests would include prolactin and luteinizing hormone.

If the volume of the ejaculate is low, a urinalysis after ejaculation is sometimes performed to assess whether the sperm has gone into the bladder. Other tests such as transrectal or scrotal ultrasound are performed if the urologist feels there may be an abnormality.

Additional tests on semen or sperm such as a DNA fragmentation test are sometimes ordered if there is a potential male factor problem. The main issue with these tests is that they cannot give the couple a clear yes-or-no answer to this question: "Will this test clearly state that I cannot get pregnant with my husband's sperm?" However, it can give percent chances, such as a low chance or high chance. If a couple decides that if there is a chance of getting pregnant with the partner's sperm they will simply go ahead, the test becomes less relevant.

Front-line perspectives

Debbi Breeden is an experienced infertility nurse. Like all of our nurses, she has direct patient contact every day. Our nurses are closest to our patients from a

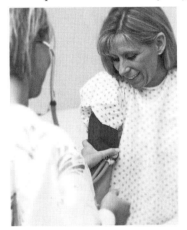

relationship standpoint. This does not mean patients don't talk with doctors and other professionals. But, day-to-day, the principal link is the nurses. Here are some of Debbi's observations.

"It seems as though once people decide they want to become parents and they've been trying with no results, they become very anxious.

"Usually when people come in for their first appointment, the anxiety level is high. Now, it's reality. This is it. We're looking at a calendar. We're making some definite plans.

"If they're a young, healthy couple, we tell them to try with unprotected intercourse for a year.

"But sometimes when we talk to them, we find factors that have interfered with the process. For example, they both may travel extensively for business and they are frequently not together at optimum times. So there are infertility issues that don't pop up even in medical textbooks.

"If we're talking to somebody who is older and they've just found that special person and they happen to be 39, we believe they shouldn't wait a full year of trying on their own. Their chances are decreasing fast. The worst scenario is somebody who didn't come to us in a timely fashion. We are definitely worried about the age of the woman.

"People should get an opinion from a board-certified infertility specialist as soon as they think they may have an issue. It doesn't mean they're going to act on it, but they're at least getting information to make intelligent decisions.

"I certainly don't try to scare people, but I definitely do make sure they understand that the medications they may go on are very powerful and that some have unpleasant side effects. I'm also very up front that there will likely be some physical pain along the way.

"There are many things that come into a final decision about what options to pursue. Nobody has to do this. It's an elective, patient-driven process. There is no so-called right answer. We want to make sure you choose a treatment plan you're both comfortable with and that you're both fully on board.

"In the final analysis, we can't help everyone. What we want to avoid is for someone to look back and second-guess their decisions. So a lot of what we do is patient education. Then our patients make the final decisions – hopefully ones they can live with for the rest of their lives no matter what those decisions may be or how the results turn out."

Frequently asked questions

Q. How long will it take to get me through the testing phase?

A. Most preliminary testing is done within one menstrual cycle. If any abnormalities are found, that will mean further tests and more time.

Q. If my husband isn't enthusiastic about going through all this, should I go ahead anyway?

A. This is a problem. However, I think it is worth having at least a consultation with an infertility specialist to gain some insight into the problem and then sharing that insight with your partner. Sometimes we can help alleviate the bleak perception that a partner may have.

Q. How much physical pain is involved with the tests?

A. The semen analysis has no pain. However, some males are uncomfortable with this. The HSG is uncomfortable, especially for patients who already have painful periods. The rest are simply blood tests.

Q. Do I have to complete all tests before getting started with trying something?

A. Generally, we recommend completing the three basic tests before starting with treatment. Those three tests are the HSG, a semen analysis, and the test for ovulation.

Q. What should I tell my extended family or close friends about what I'm doing?

A. That is a personal decision. It is interesting that some couples bring other family members to the first consult because the patient is afraid of missing information.

Q. Is it normal for people going through this to be depressed?

A. It is normal to have some anxiety and depression. However, if that escalates to a point where it interferes with your normal activities, counseling is recommended.

Q. When we're all done with the testing, will you give me a candid assessment of my chances?

A. Yes. A realistic expectation of success is important for both the couple and their doctor. The infertility specialist should lay out the facts, let the couple decide what they want to do, and then proceed with what they want. Each couple must make their own decisions. Couples ask all the time, "What are my chances, Doc?" The answer to that question is seen as good news to some and therefore worth going forward, and as bad news by others who then stop.

Patient talk

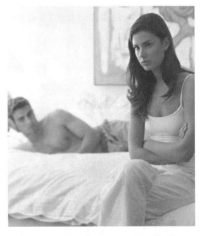

Carol and Don were married about three years when they started trying to get pregnant. Ultimately, it would take another five years for them to reach their goal. Along the way, they would switch doctors twice and experience heartache and frustration.

Says Don, "As it turned out, I needed to get checked and I was part of the problem. I had low sperm motility. I was surprised by this, but that was the diagnosis for me. We know other people who have had difficulty getting pregnant and the guys often say, 'I know it isn't me.' That's crazy. I tell them they've got to go get checked out."

Carol adds, "We started trying at the age of 27. It just didn't happen. Ultimately, we found our way to the Cleveland Clinic. We were young, we were scared, and we got frustrated. So we switched to a doctor closer to home. He had a wonderful reputation. But as it turned out, we determined that he was more female-focused than male-focused. He pushed and he prodded, but nothing happened and all the while it was costing us a lot of money.

"I remember driving home one day and the air was just taken out of us. We were both so depressed. Finally, this doctor told us we'd be lucky if we ever had one child and would most likely never have a family. That's when we took a six-month break.

"Refreshed, we went back up to Cleveland. By this time, a new procedure called ICSI (injection of one sperm directly into an egg in vitro) was gaining favor for couples like us who had a sperm-related issue. This appealed to us in particular because we wanted to reduce the potential for multiple births. For us, selective reduction of multiple embryos would never have been an option. The doctors and nurses were completely supportive of our views on selective reduction.

Don and Carol say, "Part of our denial thing was thinking we could somehow get pregnant without having to go as far as in vitro. Finally, we got to the point where we just said let's stop messing around. Let's just do it. All of our friends knew what we were doing. We weren't quiet about it at all.

"You have to have both oars in the water," says Don, "both yours and hers. You're two people. You're in your own battle. Everyone tries to help, but they're not in the battle. You are. As we learned from all the medical people, infertility is a couple's problem. Success often doesn't happen quickly. It certainly didn't for us. There's testing. There's medicine. There's waiting for the optimum time. In our case, there were plenty of failures along the way."

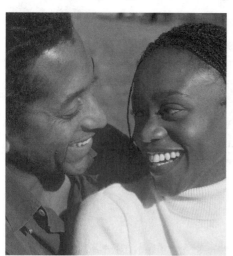

How does their story end? Two healthy boys four years apart via the ICSI procedure of IVF.

Their message? "Put your time in. You don't do this overnight. There is a lot of testing and waiting. Lose the control thing. Do everything you can to maximize your opportunities."

Summary

Both the woman and the man must be evaluated for infertility. Although many would think the woman is automatically the one with the problem, that is often not the case. There is a large population of men who are either the primary reason for infertility or at least a contributor to infertility.

There are many tests. There is a logical sequence to how they are scheduled. As one cause of infertility is eliminated, another potential cause becomes suspect.

As a certain well-known baseball player once said, "When you come to a fork in the road, take it." With infertility, there may be many forks in the road. You need to take them all. Follow where they lead. If they come to a dead end, follow another one until you get where you need to go.

Now that you have some understanding of what it takes to assess infertility issues in women and men, let's get into what it takes to address those issues. That's the subject of the next several chapters.

Chapter 5
Understanding and Fixing Female Infertility
(up to In Vitro Fertilization)

> *"Every worthwhile accomplishment, big or little,*
> *has its stages of drudgery and triumph;*
> *a beginning, a struggle, and a victory."*
> – *Anonymous*

The first step of your journey was to determine what – if any – specific issues are inhibiting your fertility.

This chapter makes the assumption that there are female issues in your case and discusses how those are most frequently addressed from a treatment standpoint up to the point of in vitro fertilization. Chapter 7 discusses IVF in some detail.

At the end of the diagnosis phase, your doctor will develop a plan to address what was found. At that point, you have to decide whether to move forward with that plan. But you need to know that whatever your doctor found must be fixed before you begin a program to address infertility.

Plain talk

Before we get into some of the details of addressing female infertility, an important point needs to be made.

One of the keys to treating infertility is to manage expectations. We help you do that. Despite that, your primary responsibility is to help manage your own expectations. Accepting that responsibility means you are willing to give yourself a reality check from time to time.

Here is your first reality check: You should be willing to come to grips with the fact that what might be termed the "fix-it" phase of infertility potentially has several associated issues.

• **Time**. Most infertility issues take time to fix. So patience is indeed a virtue. Do not look for a quick fix. If you do, there is a very good chance you will end up frustrated, disappointed, and angry.

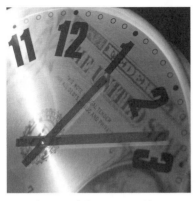

• **Discomfort**. This is a common issue with respect to either therapeutic drugs or surgery. Please understand that you are not entering a pain-free zone.

• **Money**. There are costs associated with infertility treatments. Most people, quite like you, have limited or no insurance coverage for procedures that have the sole purpose of overcoming infertility. You need to go into this with your eyes wide open from a financial standpoint. (Please see Chapter 10 on costs.)

Counterbalancing those negative factors, of course, is your positive goal – a baby.

A good, practical rule of thumb is this: As long as you believe achieving your positive goal outweighs the negative side issues that come along with it, you should keep going. But if the negative side issues take control, step back and regroup before you proceed. There are, for example, many successful case histories in which the couple took a break somewhere in the middle.

In an ideal world, it is certainly preferable to keep moving forward without interruption. But don't be afraid to take a timeout if you need one. Don't be embarrassed to raise that issue with your doctor.

At milestones along the way, ask yourself (and your spouse or partner) these three questions:

1. Are we still willing to pay the price – painfully, emotionally, financially – to try to reach our goal?

2. Are we still in agreement?

3. Do we still want a baby so much that we are willing to keep going, knowing there are no guarantees at the end of the line?

You are entering a significant medical phase when you address infertility issues.

You may think they are all about science, but that would not be correct. Infertility issues also involve key issues of the spirit: Purpose. Tenacity. Courage. Resilience.

All of those relate to managing expectations during the process. You will be much happier if you learn to do that at the outset.

Although there are no scientific studies to support this, we believe managing expectations contributes to maximizing fertility potential. It only makes sense that full focus on the goal is more helpful than half focus on the goal and half focus on all the negative stuff.

Battling your own uncertainty takes valuable, positive energy from what you are trying to accomplish. Keep your eyes on the prize and chances are you will deal with the therapeutic drug and surgery issues just fine.

Medically speaking

The most common causes of female infertility are tubal disease, problems of ovulation, and endometriosis.

Causes such as myomas/fibroids are far less common with the majority of those patients having normal fertility.

Other problems thought to play a very minor role in infertility are problems with cervical mucus and with the immune system or the blood-clotting system.

Today, a significant number of infertility cases are labeled "idiopathic," which basically means no specific cause has been identified.

Sometimes a specific cause can be found if further testing is performed, but it will not change the management of a case. Under these circumstances, a couple must decide whether they wish to undergo a test simply to know what the cause is or whether they prefer to just get on with treatment.

Ovulatory disorders

The most common cause of an ovulatory disturbance is polycystic ovary syndrome (PCOS). Other causes are overproduction of a hormone called prolactin and thyroid disease.

Polycystic ovary syndrome is one of the most common hormonal problems in women. It is estimated that one in ten women may have some form of this problem. Although the name has the word "cyst" in it, the disease manifestations do not relate to the small painless cysts that are present on the ovary. The primary manifestation relates to the disruption of the menstrual cycle and to skin and hair problems.

With PCOS, the menstrual period can be irregular or completely absent. The skin of the face and body can show signs of excess hair and acne. Patients with this syndrome have a significant health risk. They are at increased risk for cancer, diabetes, heart disease, and cholesterol problems.

The diagnosis is made when two of these criteria are present:

- No ovulatory cycles or few of those cycles.

- Elevated levels of blood male hormones (androgens) or clinical manifestation of these hormones such as acne or excessive hair (hirsutism) or thinning hair.

- An ultrasound exam showing tiny cysts on the ovaries.

The blood tests performed when this diagnosis is suspected are to exclude other causes that may be indicated with the same symptoms (such as elevated prolactin) and to confirm the diagnosis. There is a debate in the medical community about what blood tests should be performed to confirm the diagnosis of PCOS. This is because some hormones, such as luteinizing hormone secreted from the pituitary gland in the brain, are released in pulses and in varying concentrations at different times of the cycle.

The cause of PCOS has not been clearly worked out. The syndrome usually starts after the first period (menarche) with irregular periods following that. Excess body weight is not considered to have caused the disease, but excess weight does play an important role in making the syndrome worse.

Women in America with PCOS have a higher weight than comparable PCOS women in Europe. Comparison of weight at the time of important events such as high-school graduation, marriage, and the time of consultation will often show an increasing weight with more menstrual cycle problems.

The increase in fat usually is distributed around the waist so that the waist circumference is high, usually more than 35 inches. Weight loss will improve most of the metabolic problems associated with PCOS.

The cause of the syndrome is related to abnormalities in the brain (pituitary gland and hypothalamus). Insulin plays a role in this disease as well. Insulin is important for maintaining blood sugar. However, it acts together with luteinizing hormone to stimulate the ovaries to produce male hormone. The higher the woman's weight, the higher the insulin that circulates. PCOS occurs more frequently in certain families. However, no clear genetic inheritance pattern has been worked out. Some ethnic groups are at increased risk of developing diabetes if they have PCOS. These are Caribbean Hispanic, Mexican American, and African American.

It is important to be aware of the potential health problems associated with PCOS. Although the focus of this book is infertility, the other issues of PCOS should be addressed with your physician. These include an assessment of the potential for cancer of the uterus, diabetes, lipid disorders, and even sleep apnea in patients with extremes of body weight. This may mean blood tests for diabetes (oral glucose tolerance test) and fasting lipids.

The treatment of PCOS depends on what part of the syndrome we want to treat. All clinical problems of PCOS can be improved with weight loss and exercise. This includes improved fertility.

The typical medical treatment for excess hair and acne, such as an oral contraceptive or anti-androgen therapy, cannot be used in women trying to get pregnant. However, a reduction in insulin levels will both aid metabolic effects and help achieve ovulation and pregnancy. Typically, a drug such as metformin will reduce insulin resistance and consequently androgen production by the ovaries. A good website for PCOS information is supported by the Polycystic Ovarian Syndrome Association (www.pcosupport.org).

High prolactin levels and thyroid disease

A high blood prolactin level is a relatively common cause of anovulation.

The cause of the high prolactin is excessive production of the hormone by cells in the pituitary gland. The pituitary gland has different types of cells. One type of cell will produce follicle-stimulating hormone and luteinizing hormone. This excessive production of prolactin could be from a larger number of prolactin-secreting cells or a benign tumor of these cells.

Magnetic resonance imaging usually is used to assess the pituitary gland. Most patients have no specific symptoms other than disruption of the menstrual cycle. The most common non-menstrual symptoms are headaches and breast milk (galactorrhea). Visual changes and decreased libido also can occur.

Certain medications can cause an increase in prolactin. These drugs are used for gastrointestinal disorders (for example, metoclopramide) or for major psychiatric disorders (for example, antipsychotics).

Symptoms of thyroid dysfunction are often nonspecific, such as constipation, and therefore a blood test for thyroid disease should be obtained in all women with anovulation or a disrupted menstrual cycle.

There are specific drugs that will treat high prolactin levels (such as bromocriptine or carbegoline) or thyroid disease. Drugs that treat high prolactin levels can cause side effects such as nausea, vomiting, and headaches. Dizziness, fainting, and low blood pressure also can occur, but they usually resolve over time. If the menstrual cycle still is disrupted or anovulation persists after correcting this disorder, the typical ovulation induction agents discussed subsequently can be used.

Other ovulatory disturbances

Other causes of ovulatory disturbances are less common.

A primary failure in the parts of the brain (hypothalamus and pituitary gland) that control the ovaries can be the result of severe stress or weight-related disorders. For example, there are patients with severe stress from medical problems such as inflammatory bowel disease.

This "shut down" of the glands also can be the result of extreme weight loss, such as anorexia or conditions of excesses in exercise. Patients with issues such as these experience a disruption of the menstrual cycle. Treating the medical condition and regaining the weight will improve the condition and result in spontaneous ovulation. However, some patients do not have full return to normal function and ovulation induction drugs are needed.

In some cases, no cause can be found for an ovulation disorder and it is simply referred to as unexplained (idiopathic) ovulatory dysfunction.

The most controversial ovulation disorder is called a luteal phase defect. This refers to a problem in the post-ovulatory period, which is the luteal phase. This could be a problem of length, typically defined as less than eleven days. It can also be diagnosed on the basis of an endometrial biopsy.

The luteal phase has characteristic features that can be identified. The endometrial appearance changes from day to day. Each day or two has some characteristic feature that a pathologist can use to assign a post-ovulatory day. So, for example, the doctor can say that the biopsy shows the endometrium to be on day ten after ovulation.

This assignment by the doctor is correlated with the day after ovulation that the biopsy was actually done. If the biopsy date corresponds to the actual date with at most a two-day difference, we call the biopsy "in phase." If there is consistently more than a two-day difference, the endometrium is termed "out of phase" and diagnostic of a luteal phase defect.

The main problem with this diagnosis is the test. First, the accuracy of the endometrial biopsy has been questioned. Second, many fertile women with children have luteal phase defects. This questions the relevance of this diagnosis.

There are several other problems with the test. The test needs to be repeated in two subsequent cycles – two biopsies – to be valid. Few women will submit to this. Rather, they simply request treatment.

The frequency of this disorder has diminished with increasing sophistication of the test procedure. Previously, a biopsy was done just before a period and the date of the biopsy based on the time of the next period. That is, to determine ovulation, we counted back fourteen days from the first day of the period and assigned that day as ovulation. However, we now know that this is inaccurate.

Today, luteinizing hormone urine kits determine ovulation and then a biopsy is performed in the mid-luteal phase (day ten to twelve) with precise dating. A biopsy then is repeated in a subsequent cycle. Using this method, luteal phase defect is found uncommonly.

Ovulation induction

The drug regimens for ovulation induction can be used with most disorders of anovulation (failure to ovulate). However, for patients with high prolactin levels or thyroid disease, the underlying medical problem should be corrected first. Treating the problem may solve the anovulatory disorder.

There are several classes of ovulation induction drugs.

The first are pills such as clomiphene citrate that act on certain areas in the brain, especially the hypothalamus. This gland senses a low estrogen level and then sends a signal to the other gland in the brain – the pituitary – to release the follicle-stimulating hormone to stimulate the ovary to produce an egg.

The production of an egg can be monitored by ultrasound or it can be indirectly confirmed with either a urine test for luteinizing hormone or a blood test for progesterone.

An egg may not necessarily release on its own. Under those circumstances, an additional medication called hCG (human chorionic gonadotropin) is necessary. This is an injection. Ovulation will occur about thirty-six hours later.

The side effects of clomiphene citrate are hot flashes, headache, and abdominal discomfort. These drugs also can cause multiple births. That risk is estimated to be between 8 and 13 percent. Visual disturbances can occur that may require discontinuing the drug. Mood swings are quite common. The drug also causes the cervical mucus to be drier and the endometrial lining to become thinner. A thin lining may not allow subsequent implantation of an embryo. If the cervical mucus is thicker, inseminations that bypass the cervix may be necessary.

Typically, we start at a low dose and increase until ovulation occurs. (If a patient does not respond to a dose such as 150 mg, it is unlikely she will respond to a higher dose.) Then the patient is maintained on that dose for about six cycles. The ovulation rate is usually 70 percent and the pregnancy rate 35 percent.

Even if the cervical mucus is fine, inseminations are also performed if pregnancy has not occurred after three cycles at an ovulatory dose. If ovulation is not induced with clomiphene citrate or if pregnancy does not occur despite proper ovulation, it is time for the next step.

Most infertility specialists believe that no more than six months of an ovulatory dose of clomiphene citrate should be used. Overweight women have a higher chance of not ovulating with clomiphene. The discrepancy between ovulation (70 percent) and pregnancy rate (35 percent) is attributed to the anti-estrogenic effects that cause dry cervical mucus and a thin uterine lining. Insemination will help the dry cervical mucus problem.

The next type of drug is called gonadotropin. A gonadotropin called hCG is used to trigger the release of an egg. The normal cycle luteinizing hormone is the actual trigger for release of the egg. The hormone hCG is produced by the placenta. However, the similarities in chemical structure between LH and hCG have allowed the use of hCG. These are synthetic or urine-derived products.

Other gonadotropins – follicle-stimulating hormone (FSH) and luteinizing hormone (LH) – stimulate the production of eggs directly in the ovary. These are injectable drugs. Some are synthetic drugs and are not derived from the urine of menopausal women while others are derived from the urine of menopausal women. These drugs are potent and are associated with high pregnancy rates.

FSH is the most important gonadotropin to stimulate egg production. Many recent formulations have only FSH. Others have a combination of both LH and FSH. In patients who are anovulatory, the starting dose is usually 50 to 75 IU and is increased after that.

Close monitoring with ultrasound and blood tests is required. These drugs can have serious side effects, including an increase in multiple births and excessive stimulation of the ovaries. Mood swings and bloating also can occur. The cycles with these drugs may cause an excessive number of eggs, which can result in cancellation of the cycle by withholding hCG and abstaining from sexual intercourse. The typical length of treatment is three cycles.

These ovulation drugs are not associated with increased risk of birth defects. However, clomiphene citrate is still detectable in the blood one month after finishing the medication. So it is present in small doses when pregnancy is achieved.

Infertile women are at an increased risk of ovarian cancer, and achieving a pregnancy will decrease the risk. It is unclear whether the ovulation drugs increase that risk. Most specialists believe that the studies do not support the major risk with these drugs. On the other hand, it is prudent to use them only when indicated and for limited periods.

In patients with PCOS, which is the most common cause of anovulation, other medications have been found to be helpful.

The first is a drug that is also used for diabetes, called metformin. We know that weight loss will induce ovulation. The weight loss probably acts by decreasing insulin resistance, a common finding in PCOS women. Metformin is an insulin-lowering drug. The dose is usually 1,500 to 2,000 mg per day. The main side effects are gastrointestinal such as diarrhea. Beginning this medication at a low dose and increasing it gradually help prevent this.

Typically, the drug is given alone at first to see whether ovulation can be induced. This usually is apparent by the restoration of a normal menstrual cycle. Insulin-lowering therapies are effective even without insulin resistance. Metformin appears to have a synergistic effect with clomiphene. Together, they work better than either does alone. It also appears that miscarriage rates and the frequency of gestational diabetes are decreased with the use of these drugs.

Another class of drugs, called aromatase inhibitors, has been recently evaluated for ovulation induction. These drugs also act on the hypothalamus in the brain to cause a release of FSH from the pituitary gland. They have no direct interaction with estrogen receptors and therefore should not have a negative effect on the cervical mucus or uterine lining. So far, letrozole is the most widely tested. The method of taking the drug is similar to clomiphene. This class of drugs usually does not persist in the body as long as clomiphene. Also, multiple births are thought to occur less frequently with letrozole. The manufacturer of letrozole does not recommend its use as a fertility drug.

There is a surgical treatment for inducing ovulation called "ovarian drilling." Although somewhat effective, it may result in scar tissue formation that can decrease fertility. Ovarian drilling done during a laparoscopy requires general anesthesia and there are always surgical risks associated with that. However, ovarian drilling may be an option after all other medical therapy has been tried without achieving a pregnancy.

Superovulation or controlled ovarian hyperstimulation is the term used when these drugs are given to women who already ovulate normally. The idea is that these drugs may correct some subtle ovulation defect or simply increase the number of eggs available for fertilization. The pregnancy rate with clomiphene and insemination in couples with no specific cause of infertility is approximately 8 to 10 percent per cycle of trying. If drugs such as FSH are used with insemination, the pregnancy rate is double. The starting dose is usually 150 IU. You should be aware that there are increased risks of multiple births with ovarian hyperstimulation.

Endometriosis

Endometriosis is a chronic inflammatory disease that can cause periodic or sustained pelvic pain and infertility in women. It is characterized by the presence of endometrial glands that line the cavity outside the uterus. A disease found in all ethnic groups, its precise origin is unknown.

There are many components of this disease that disrupt the immune system. Although not considered a hereditary disease, it is more frequent in some family groups and has a genetic component.

With endometriosis, menstruation occurs upward into the abdomen at the same time as vaginally. Normally, the body can clear these glands from the abdomen. However, if there is a dysfunction in the peritoneal clearance mechanism or if there are intrinsic features of the glands that allow it to escape clearance, these glands will persist. An inflammatory response will then occur that may result in scar tissue, which is very unhelpful to fertility.

Environmental pollutants are involved in this disease. However, their precise contribution is unclear. Animal research data clearly points to the fact that dioxins or dioxin-like pollutants such as polychlorinated biphenyls can cause endometriosis. These pollutants can disrupt the hormonal and immune mechanism of the body and are often referred to as "endocrine disruptors." These wastes are found in food.

However, endometriosis is a complex disease that cannot be attributed solely to this exposure. For example, there was a factory explosion in Seveso, Italy, in 1976 that resulted in an extremely high exposure to dioxin. Women under 30 years of age were followed for decades. The increase in endometriosis risk was marginal. Yet a similar study in Belgium reported a higher risk increase.

The diagnosis of endometriosis is suspected in women with painful periods (dysmenorrhea), painful sexual intercourse (dyspareunia), and chronic pelvic pain. This disease is definitely associated with infertility. However, patients with endometriosis may achieve pregnancy without intervention.

Endometriosis can be confirmed only by laparoscopy. Blood tests and ultrasound cannot make the diagnosis of endometriosis. The presence of a persistent ovarian cyst will make us suspect its presence. The disease is classified at surgery as a Stage 1, 2, 3, or 4. This is based on a special scoring system. It is important to stage the disease so that a precise decision on prognosis can be made.

It is clear that the surgical treatment of endometriosis will improve fertility. The early stages of disease may show a doubling of pregnancy rates, but that is still less than for fertile women. The more advanced disease also will have an improvement in fertility, but the surgery is technically challenging.

Medical therapy that suppresses the menstrual cycle, like the birth-control pill or a gonadotropin-releasing hormone agonist that works quite well in controlling the pain symptoms, does not improve fertility. However, ovulation induction drugs and in vitro fertilization will improve fertility rates.

The advantage of surgery is that pregnancy can subsequently occur spontaneously without the use of fertility drugs. The disadvantage is that surgery requires time to work. Therefore in women of older reproductive age, over 35 for example, it may be wiser to proceed more quickly to fertility drugs or IVF.

Tubal disease and pelvic adhesions

The most common cause of infertility is blocked tubes that result from previous infection.

Sexually transmitted diseases cause infection and scar-tissue formation. The severity of the disease is quite variable and ranges from simple adhesions with preservation of tubal structure to the extreme with maximal tubal destruction and severe adhesions. An X-ray or an HSG can usually detect this problem. However, the definitive test is a laparoscopy.

During a laparoscopy procedure, the entire pelvis can be viewed and the severity of disease assessed. If the disease of the tubes is in fact severe, there may be a dilatation of the tubes called a hydrosalpinx. This problem is not repairable and it may decrease the fertility rates from IVF. Therefore, removal of the damaged tube is recommended.

If, on the other hand, damage to the tube is mild to moderate, repair is possible. Repair for the tube can be performed by laparoscopy. In this way, recovery from the surgery is relatively quick. Pregnancy rates are good, and a couple is given a chance for a spontaneous pregnancy. The main complication of this procedure is the increased risk of ectopic pregnancy with the repair.

Ectopic pregnancy is the implantation of a pregnancy outside the uterus, usually in the uterine tube. If left untreated, the tube can rupture, causing hemorrhage and even death. However, the vast majority of ectopic pregnancies can be treated successfully with medical therapy as long as the problem is discovered quickly. The medication used to accomplish that is called methotrexate and is given as an injection.

Surgery is sometimes required to remove an ectopic pregnancy. If there is rupture or severe tubal damage, the tube may need to be removed as well.

Most ectopic pregnancies occur spontaneously without tubal surgery. It is thought that there must be some underlying tubal damage that restricts the movement of the embryo inside the tube and prevents it from entering the uterus. However, after surgical repair of a damaged tube, the risk of ectopic pregnancy is increased.

The diagnosis of ectopic pregnancy should be suspected when a pregnancy occurs in any patient undergoing infertility treatment. This diagnosis is made with serial blood tests that show an inappropriate rise in the pregnancy hormone hCG. Additionally, a vaginal ultrasound is performed to confirm that a pregnancy is in the uterus rather than the uterine tube. Scar tissue from previous surgery can involve the tube and cause infertility. For example, a ruptured appendix or surgery for inflammatory bowel disease can cause severe adhesions. An evaluation of the severity of the disease will determine whether it is possible to repair the tube or it is better to proceed directly to IVF.

Fibroids/myomas

Fibroids are benign tumors often found in or on the uterus.

Fibroids are more commonly seen in certain ethnic groups such as African Americans. They may occur in different parts of the uterus. Most fibroids are small and do not cause any problems. The mere presence of a fibroid of whatever size is not an indication for removal. However, if a patient is interested in having children, the impact of the size of the fibroid on a pregnancy should be discussed with an obstetrician.

Some patients have a menstrual problem that is caused by a fibroid. The management of the menstrual disorder caused by a fibroid is usually surgery. It is uncommon that a hysterectomy is required to treat fibroids.

Normally, removal of the fibroids is accomplished by a surgical procedure called a myomectomy. An experienced surgeon should be able to remove the fibroids even if many involve the uterus.

Fibroids that occur in the cavity of the uterus usually can be treated by hysteroscopy, a procedure where a tiny camera is placed through the cervix. Using this camera, small instruments are passed into the cavity and the fibroid is removed. This procedure is the ideal approach in all women, especially those who are interested in achieving a pregnancy.

In some women who are not interested in future fertility, a radiologic procedure called embolization may be an option. It is very effective in managing the menstrual problem associated with fibroids. Although pregnancies have occurred after this procedure, there are insufficient data yet on pregnancy outcomes. Preliminary information suggests there may be increased pregnancy complications resulting from this procedure.

If surgery is indicated, there is a potential that it can be performed by laparoscopy. Laparoscopy as an outpatient procedure offers the potential for a speedier recovery than open surgery (laparotomy). There are limitations on the size and location of the fibroid that can be removed by laparoscopy.

The most feared complication after myomectomy is uterine rupture during pregnancy – especially during labor. The surgeon must ensure that when the fibroid is removed, the defect on the uterus is appropriately closed to withstand labor.

The relationship between fibroids and infertility is not clear. Thus, removal of fibroids just for fertility reasons is not routine. If there is a distortion of the uterine cavity documented by X-ray, ultrasound, or hysteroscopy, consideration is given to removing the fibroid primarily for fertility reasons. Usually, if there is no distortion of the cavity, fibroid surgery is not necessary.

The potential of a fibroid to cause problems during pregnancy should be discussed with an obstetrician before proceeding with pregnancy. If surgery is to be done for primarily infertility reasons, a complete investigation into other causes of infertility should be done first.

If a fibroid is removed, complications can occur after surgery. The most common are fever, infection, and bleeding that may require a blood transfusion. Scar tissue also may form, which actually can cause infertility. Rarely is a hysterectomy required.

Premature ovarian failure

Premature ovarian failure (POF) refers to the inability of the ovary to function at an early age (defined as less than 40).

This inability to function may be the result of depletion of the follicles that contain the eggs or inability of these follicles to respond and ovulate. The causes of this problem can be genetic or autoimmune.

The diagnosis is made when an adult woman consults with a physician because her menstrual period is absent or comes infrequently. The blood test for follicle-stimulating hormone is elevated as it is in a menopausal woman. The younger the age this occurs, such as in adolescents, the higher the chance that we are dealing with a genetic cause. Therefore, in women under 30, we order a chromosomal analysis.

A frequent cause of POF is an autoimmune process similar to thyroid disease. Autoimmune glandular failure occurs frequently in women. Auto-antibodies occur against the cells in the ovary. However, there are no good tests available that can measure these antibodies routinely.

Having the antibody does not mean that POF will occur. Likewise, just because somebody does not have the antibody does not mean that POF is not due to an autoimmune phenomenon. A biopsy is not recommended to prove there is an inflammation in the ovary. The diagnosis is made by a blood test.

Several other autoimmune diseases occur with POF. The most common are antibodies against the adrenal gland, the thyroid gland, and the pancreas. Patients can develop conditions such as hypothyroidism, diabetes mellitus, and adrenal failure (called Addison's disease). Therefore, tests should be performed to exclude these diseases. Although these conditions can be treated, patients do not respond to any form of fertility treatment currently offered. The only treatment available is through a donor egg program. However, the prognosis is not totally bleak. Although there is no specific treatment, approximately 8 percent of women with such disorders can in fact ovulate spontaneously and get pregnant.

Since the symptoms of early ovarian failure are similar to menopause, therapy to prevent the consequences of low estrogen such as osteoporosis should be started.

Infertility and the cancer patient

The excellent rate of survival of childhood cancers and the occurrence of certain cancers like breast cancer in reproductive-age women have brought to the fore the problems of infertility in cancer survivors.

The best approach, of course, is prevention of ovarian damage before it occurs. Both the ovaries and testes are very sensitive to chemotherapy and radiation therapy. The age of the woman at the time of treatment as well as the total dose of chemo or radiation therapy will determine the degree of damage. The younger the age of the patient when she receives the treatment, the more resistant her ovaries are to treatment.

If radiation will be the only treatment for her cancer, a discussion with the oncologist or gynecologist about moving the ovaries out of the way should occur. This procedure, called ovarian transposition, can be performed by laparoscopy on an outpatient basis and permits a rapid recovery. The reported rates of success are variable. However, modern surgical procedures have made this technique more feasible. Furthermore, this technique has a proven track record of results that other techniques do not have.

Chemotherapy damage to the ovary is dependent on the dose and type of agent. Alkylating agents are the most toxic. However, not all patients exposed to these agents develop ovarian failure. A discussion about this with your oncologist and infertility specialist is important. One option is to use a gonadotropin-releasing hormone agonist to try to suppress the ovary and protect it against damage. This approach, too, is controversial. However, there is minimal toxicity with such a hormonal drug, and these drugs may also prevent some of the menstrual problems that occur with chemotherapy. Such a drug therapy is simple to start since it is an intramuscular injection monthly or every three months.

Another possibility is to proceed to in vitro fertilization before the chemotherapy. In this way the ovaries are stimulated, and the eggs are retrieved, fertilized, and stored by cryopreservation. This technique works quite well, but it takes at least two weeks to accomplish. The main limitations are time and the need for a partner.

Understandably, oncologists are hesitant to delay chemotherapy for this period of time. If this procedure is used in women with breast cancer, it is important to use drugs that do not excessively increase estrogens, as with the use of a class of drugs called aromatase inhibitors. If there is no partner, an attempt can be made to freeze (cryopreserve) the eggs. Although this technology has poorer results than embryo freezing, dozens of pregnancies have been reported.

There is also potential to freeze ovarian tissue. The ovarian tissue is obtained by an outpatient procedure called a laparoscopy and the tissue frozen. However, very few pregnancies from cryopreserved ovarian tissue have been reported, and the procedure is deemed experimental.

In women with gynecological malignancies, a conservative approach that does not remove all the reproductive organs may be possible. For example, in certain cervical cancers, only the cervix needs to be removed. In endometrial cancers, high-dose hormonal therapy may save the uterus. In early-stage ovarian cancer, perhaps one ovary only can be removed.

The most important concept is that there are potential choices. If fertility is still an option, these choices should be discussed. A good support group for cancer patients can be found at www.fertilehope.org.

Front-line perspectives

Suzy Pare is a longtime nurse-practitioner in our OB/GYN section.

"A lot of the women who come to us are older in terms of fertility – in their mid to late 30s – and they have long ago taken control of their lives to get where they are today. They try to take control of their infertility issue, too. They find there isn't any control to be had in the conventional sense. With infertility, you gain a measure of control by asking good questions and doing what you have to do. You need to be positive and forward-thinking but also realistic about what you can expect based on your test results.

"They are hopeful. They are excited to feel they are now getting somewhere at last. But often they are also depressed and angry. We see big ranges of behavior. Some women come in and feel the only way they can get what they want is to push hard. But then they discover we really will spend time with them on the phone and answer their questions, and many of them settle down and become more positive.

"Sometimes people just fade away because the whole thing is just too much for them. They feel it's too slow or too expensive or they're simply not willing to do what we suggest. Some will come back a year later in a different frame of mind. Some find other treatments or pursue adoption.

"Being well organized is really, really important. Both parties need to be able to look ahead and schedule their time. This is particularly true with respect to business travel. If the husband is traveling at a pivotal time, we can freeze the sperm. But if the wife is on the road at that key time, that's a big problem. So it really helps to focus and plan your life ahead of time to do what you need to do.

"It's not at all uncommon for females to come to us who are already on antidepressants. Sometimes it's hard to know if this is chronic depression or situational depression related to infertility. We have a couple of therapists on our hospital staff who specialize in working with these issues for infertile couples. Our therapists have really helped them.

"People need coping skills. Some think if we suggest a therapist that we think they're nuts. That's wrong. We're not saying you're nuts. We're saying this is hard and you need help to get through this.

"At the end, some people meet their goal and some don't. Regardless, it's very, very important for couples to always be able to look back and know they did everything they could. That might not mean everything that is available. It means everything they're compatible with. In that context, success is feeling at peace with yourself."

Frequently asked questions

Q. I know you'll do a plan for us. What are the important things I need to know about that plan?

A. You need to consider the risks, benefits, and outcomes of each option.

Q. Is there more than one approach you can take to my issue?

A. There is always more than one option for infertility treatment. The decision is based on what risks (medical and financial) the couple is willing to take to achieve the outcome. For example, with clomiphene and inseminations, we can expect a 10 percent pregnancy rate in a 30-year-old woman after one attempt. With IVF, the pregnancy rate is over 50 percent. The risks and costs are higher with the latter choice, but so is the potential outcome.

Q. How long will it take to get me fixed up so we can get on with getting pregnant?

A. There really is no good answer. It simply depends on the problem.

Q. What are the best things for me to be doing to help you make me fertile?

A. Follow the general principles outlined in the chapter about preventing infertility (Chapter 3).

Q. Why does all this take so long?

A. Except with use of sophisticated technology, it takes a long time because pregnancy rates per month are low in humans. In addition, the implementation of a treatment plan can be delayed for personal reasons or simply because of the logistics of implementing a plan.

Q. What do I do if I hit a sudden problem or have an important new question?

A. Usually, the nurse on call can answer your question. Of course, you have direct access to your doctor by phone, e-mail, or in-person consultation.

Q. Will I have to miss work if I need surgery?

A. That depends on the treatment. For most procedures, surgery typically requires a commitment of seven to ten days. You should also know that ovulation induction may require frequent visits for ultrasound exams or blood tests.

Patient talk

Mary Ann has a complex medical history. Chronic pain. Multiple medical issues. Difficult choices along the way.

And she also has a happy ending: three fine-looking, active, normal children.

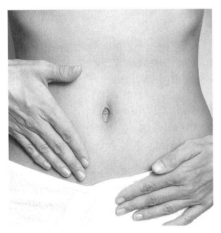

Her journey started with a gynecologist in 1999 for pain issues, not infertility problems. "The pain would come out of nowhere. I couldn't even stand up. It was a stabbing, grabbing pain that would last for a couple of hours," she says.

The diagnosis was endometriosis. The recommendation was abdominal surgery.

She went to another doctor for a second opinion late that year. He performed a laparoscopy procedure. "He told me I was such a mess inside that he wanted to do a full hysterectomy," Mary Ann says.

"My next step was to do my own research on the web. I believe everyone needs to be their own advocate, that everyone needs to educate themselves. This is how I found my other doctor. The information on him indicated that he had laparoscopy as one of his specialties.

"When I got to him, we knew my tubes were flowing because of the earlier tests. But he said the only way to figure out my situation for sure was to do another laparoscopy. He did that and diagnosed fibroids. I just had so many, and they were twisted around and causing great pain. It didn't happen every day, but it happened frequently. I also had a lot of adhesions without a history of STDs. Endometriosis in my case was not a big problem. He did surgery on the fibroids and freed up as many adhesions as possible. He said there was really no reason I couldn't get pregnant."

Mary Ann is in a committed partnership with a woman named Lynne. They wanted to have children. In this instance, they worked with a sperm bank to select a donor. This was a rigorous process for them. "We looked at my family history, our culture, and ethnicity. Because I was going to be the biological parent, we also looked at my family history and knew we did not want to duplicate certain things. We were concerned about allergies, learning disabilities, a history of cancer, and some other issues.

"It had been suggested that we use a donor with medium skin and dark eyes. I said no. I wanted somebody with eyes that match mine. It will be important to the children someday when they look at me as the biological parent that they see something that tells them they are okay because they can see where they come from.

"The donor I ended up choosing had what you might call a 'boy-next-door' description. But you really don't know who it is. You just look at the facts on a piece of paper. Ultimately, you have to trust them. We did choose a donor with some shared ethnicity to Lynne.

"I did a series of inseminations over nine months with no luck. We then moved up to IVF. They were able to harvest fourteen eggs, of which twelve became embryos. I was 37 years old at the time, so they implanted three of the twelve. Two of those took on the first try, and we now have twins, a boy and a girl.

"The other nine embryos were frozen and set aside. Six months after the birth of the twins, we wanted to try again. Six of the frozen embryos survived the cryopreservation process. We set a date, and they thawed out four. None of those made it. But we still had two left. They ended up implanting the two, and that is how we have our other little boy." (Although this child is 16 months younger than his siblings from the standpoint of birth age, he is also their triplet since he came from the same batch of embryos.)

Mary Ann did not have a smooth pregnancy the first time. She had a major scare that she had miscarried just prior to the twelve-week point and did not get reassurance that had not happened until the twenty-fourth week. She spent the last eight weeks of her first pregnancy in bed. Neither did she have an easy time giving birth. Mary Ann had a significant internal bleeding issue resulting from the birth process. On the other hand, the second pregnancy and birth were essentially problem-free.

Says Mary Ann, "It can be a long road, exhausting not only for yourself, but also for the people who care about you – your spouse, your parents, and others in your family. It affects everybody. But at the same time, you're going through it alone. And there is a lot of discomfort. The drugs do give you mood swings and make you hormone-crazy. You have to maintain your sanity and find some way to keep a center."

Her best advice? "Unless you get your information from your doctor or a medical journal, be very cautious about what you read and hear."

Another lesson to be learned from a parenting relationship such as this one is to have estate planning in order (including living wills) – especially because any medical procedures carry some element of risk. You want to make sure your children are cared for and that your partner can make decisions.

Summary

You don't need to remember all the medical terms. What you do need to remember is that there are many different approaches to infertility and that you have to have enough patience to get to the one that will work best for you.

There is "no free lunch" when it comes to infertility treatment. It takes time. You can expect some pain – physical and/or emotional. And there are hard financial costs associated with this treatment as well. Be realistic. Manage your own expectations.

If you need to call a timeout somewhere in the process, know that others before you have done that same thing.

Surround yourself with positive people. Be positive yourself. Think good thoughts.

Chapter 6
Understanding and Fixing Male Infertility
(up to In Vitro Fertilization)

"The superior man makes the difficulty to be overcome his first interest; success comes only later."

– Confucius

This chapter examines how we address the most common male factors that are so frequently either the root cause of or a contributing factor to infertility.

Plain talk

"Okay, Mr. Smith, it's time for a reality check. You've got a problem. We need to fix it if you want to reach your goal."

Those are words no man ever wants to hear.

But those words are part of the emotional roller coaster many couples encounter

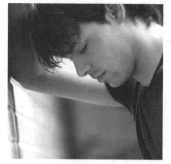

when they begin to address their infertility issues.

If you want to cross the finish line a winner, you must learn to live with the daily ups and downs of infertility. Recognizing and accepting that challenge will be helpful as you deal with it.

There are significant advantages for couples when a urologist addressing male factor infertility is an integral member of the total infertility medical practice as compared to being independent from that practice. Coordinated plans and effective communication offer excellent potential for good results.

Many of the infertility issues women face can be addressed successfully with drug therapies. This is less so with male infertility factor. Drug therapy is not the answer for most men. Correctable causes of male infertility are usually treated with surgery rather than with drug therapy.

Every male infertility issue relates to sperm – its quantity, shape, and strength of movement. Ideally, the evaluation is thorough enough to isolate the cause of a low or absent sperm count or poor-quality sperm. A "fix" is available for some of these men. This may include surgery, medication, or manipulation of the sperm to enhance the chance of fertilizing an egg.

So, men, managing your expectations means dealing with the possibility of a few visits to a urologist trained in male infertility. Then, depending on what is found, you may experience either a trial of medication, a surgical procedure, or isolating the best sperm possible to be used for insemination or in vitro fertilization.

In the previous chapter, "Addressing and Fixing Female Infertility," we cautioned that couples look carefully at three key issues.

The first was the issue of time. As with female infertility, fixing male infertility is not like flipping a light switch. It will likely take some time for the sperm to normalize, if it does at all. Typically, it takes three to six months to appreciate whether improvement will occur.

The second was discomfort. If you have to have surgery, most of the time that is not something that will require a huge incision. But it is surgery. All surgery can cause some discomfort and require a period of recovery (often brief) before you are back to normal. Manage your expectations on that issue as well.

The third was money. Again, you are referred to Chapter 10 for discussion of this important issue. In most but not all cases, insurance coverage will be tied to whether the evaluation, tests, or any procedure are deemed medically necessary and/or related to another illness versus strictly associated with the issue of infertility. Understand your own situation. Unless you are one of the fortunate few, you will be out of pocket for some or all of the testing and procedures intended to overcome male infertility factors.

It is important to understand that there are millions of men with infertility issues. These sperm issues have no impact on your ability to have a normal and happy sex life. But they may have an impact on your ability to father a child.

So if being a dad is at the top of your priority list, you must participate fully in the process. If that's the goal you have set for yourself, that is the goal we have for you.

So here's what you may expect if you own part or all of the infertility problem in your house.

Medically speaking

The concept of male infertility is not necessarily an easy one to define.

It is, of course, clear that if there are no sperm, the male is infertile.

However, often the counts are lower than the normal range that the lab gives. A poor semen analysis does not automatically mean infertility. We cannot say that a man with a sperm count of 18 million/ml is infertile. Nor can we definitely say that a man with a count above 20 million/ml is fertile.

What we can say is that in a group of males, the lower the motile sperm count (motility equals movement), the lower the spontaneous pregnancy rates. The reason for the variation is because of the different fertility potential of the partner. Clearly, a more fertile woman may be able to compensate somewhat for low semen quality just as a man with high-quality sperm in his ejaculate may compensate for a woman who has less than optimal fertility.

There are many other tests available for semen than those discussed in this chapter. However, many of these tests have poor predictive value. For this reason, the more sophisticated tests are not commonly used by infertility doctors.

Male factor infertility can be divided into three distinct categories:

- Problems associated with production of sperm.
- Problems associated with transporting the sperm from the testicles to the vagina.
- Problems associated with fertilizing an egg.

Production of normal sperm

The production of normal sperm is complex and requires communication between parts of the brain (hypothalamus and pituitary gland) and the testicles.

The testicles have two functions:

1. To produce male hormone (testosterone).

2. To produce sperm.

These two functions are somewhat separate in the male. For example, a man can have no sperm at all but still have normal levels of male hormone. However, a certain amount of male hormone is necessary for sperm production. In women, of course, hormone production (estrogen) is tied to the presence of eggs. If there are no eggs, there will be very little estrogen production from the ovary.

Abnormalities of these glands in a man's brain can cause the testicles to function improperly. Typically when that occurs, patients have obvious symptoms. One instance would be that patients who are born with these problems may not subsequently go into puberty. Others will develop testicle failure (hypogonadal male) from a glandular problem in the brain, such as a benign pituitary tumor. These males may complain of markedly decreased libido. This tumor can produce a hormone called prolactin, which can be detected in a blood test and an imaging study (MRI) of the brain.

The testicles produce the sperm in a specialized area called seminiferous tubules. Sperm in this area are not mature. However, in some cases of male infertility, this is the only sperm available. The sperm become mature in the epididymis, a coiled structure behind the testicles that stores sperm.

The sperm then have to travel through these ducts to be ejaculated. These ducts can be obstructed or absent. During a vasectomy, one of these ducts – the vas deferens – is occluded. The ejaculate is made up of sperm and secretions from glands such as the prostate. Ejaculated sperm can live about two days in the female.

The most common problems that cause male infertility are these:

- Idiopathic (unknown) in 30 to 50 percent of cases.

- Varicocele (testicles with varicose veins).

- Obstruction of the ducts that transport sperm from the testicles, as with a vasectomy.

- Genetic disorders.

- Hormone abnormalities or imbalances.

A low sperm count is referred to as oligospermia; no sperm at all is called azoospermia.

When a low sperm count is found, we usually proceed to some other tests as well as a detailed physical exam of the man by a male infertility specialist – typically a urologist.

Varicoceles

The presence of a varicocele is one of the most common causes of infertility and low sperm counts, poor motility, or a high number of abnormally shaped sperm.

A varicocele is a dilation of the veins that ascend from the testicles. Those veins drain into the testicular vein that goes toward the large vein in the abdomen. These veins surround the testicular artery. The artery brings blood to the testicle, and the vein drains the testicles.

The veins in the scrotum that surround the artery cool the blood going to the testicles. This is important because the temperature in the testicles is lower than body temperature. The important concept in this is that the dilated veins disrupt this cooling mechanism and alter testicular function. This is clearly not helpful to fertility.

The way this cooling mechanism disrupts testicular function is the subject of some debate. The main problem in attributing the infertility problem solely to the varicocele is that the majority of men with this condition are still fertile. However, it is possible but unproven that over time a varicocele may lead to deterioration of fertility. Therefore, many urologists specializing in infertility recommend repair to avoid further damage to the testicle. It is important to point out here that varicoceles do not have an impact on general health.

The diagnosis of a varicocele is made initially by physical examination and is subsequently confirmed by ultrasound. Most infertility specialists agree that varicoceles detected only by ultrasound are not clinically important to the infertility problem. Although varicoceles usually affect all semen parameters, they also can cause isolated problems such as sperm shape (morphology) issues.

The decision to repair or not to repair a varicocele is dependent on several variables. The most important is the fertility status of the partner. If the woman's fertility is significantly impaired, intervention may be required to optimize the results for a female problem. Sometimes a female problem cannot be adequately treated. In that case, there is less reason to treat a varicocele. For example, if IVF is indicated to treat blocked tubes in the woman and there is sufficient sperm in the man's ejaculate, most couples may choose to forgo repair of a varicocele.

If there are no female problems, the couple must also accept the interval that may be required to achieve a pregnancy. Improvement in semen parameters may take six to nine months and then they should attempt pregnancy for another six to nine months before proceeding with alternatives. So this points out once again the need for patience and appropriate expectations for infertility patients.

Repairs for a varicocele can be performed by radiologic surgery or microsurgical repair. Each procedure does have some risk. Generally, recovery is quite rapid with both. Most men are able to return to work in three to four days and full activity within seven to ten days.

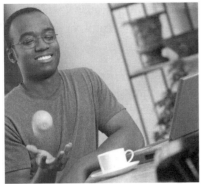

Varicocele repair will improve semen parameters in most cases. The improvement in pregnancy rates is still the subject of much debate by infertility specialists. The main advantage is that a patient can attempt a spontaneous pregnancy without the risks of multiple births that are typically seen with most assisted reproductive technology such as in vitro fertilization. Furthermore, there are risks with assisted reproductive technology, such as ovarian hyperstimulation, that are not present if the decision is to proceed with intervention in the male.

Unknown oligospermia

Many cases of low sperm counts do not have a clear-cut origin and are referred to as unknown or idiopathic. After proper medical examination and investigation, there may not be any specific treatment modality. Over time, there has been a general trend toward reduced sperm counts in many countries. This has been attributed to widespread use of pesticides and other environmental pollutants.

The effects of these pollutants are thought to be responsible for a global increase in testicular cancer. For example, men from Denmark have the lowest sperm counts and the highest risk of testicular cancer in the world.

The contaminants that have raised the most suspicion are pesticides, cigarette smoke, and dioxins.

There also is a phenomenon called oxidative stress that affects sperm. This involves oxygen molecules that can damage DNA, the genetic component of a cell. There are many other health effects of oxidative stress such as heart disease. It is for this reason that many specialists recommend that men take antioxidants such as vitamins C and E. However, there are no studies to show that this regimen actually improves fertility and therefore it is recommended that couples proceed to treatment.

There are no data to support the use of nutritional supplements except what is reasonable for a healthy lifestyle. It is important to reiterate here that the nutritional supplements that are supposed to improve "fertility" have not been proved to work. Further, the expense of these supplements can be prohibitive.

Very low sperm count can mean that a genetic problem is a cause of infertility. Because of that, men should be tested as described below because of the potential to pass this genetic problem on to their male children.

Severe male factor infertility requires in vitro fertilization or donor insemination. Mild forms of male factor infertility can be treated with insemination.

Insemination

Insemination is the process by which ejaculated sperm is placed artificially in the female reproductive tract.

The sperm can be placed on the cervix or inside the cavity of the uterus (intrauterine insemination or IUI). Intrauterine insemination implies that ejaculated semen is prepared in a specific way that allows it to be placed directly into the uterine cavity. This process removes substances from seminal fluid that may cause uterine contractions, such as prostaglandins. Fresh, unprocessed sperm should not be placed in the uterus.

Donor sperm insemination is performed when the husband has no sperm or when there is no male partner. Donor insemination is also an option for a couple when the sperm parameters are such that the only effective medical treatment is in vitro fertilization and the couple has chosen not to proceed with IVF. Some couples, for financial, religious, or other reasons, feel that IVF is not for them.

Donor insemination is also used for couples where the male has a genetic defect that the couple does not wish to pass on. Finally, it is used when the man has a sexually transmitted disease such as HIV.

Donor insemination programs have rigorous standards. The male screening is detailed and involves screening for psychological problems, STDs, and genetic disorders.

Donors should be healthy males under 40. The sperm is frozen and quarantined for at least six months and released only if retesting of the male shows no evidence of an STD. Only frozen semen should be used.

Typically a recipient couple undergoes psychological evaluation before proceeding through this process. They also undergo screening for STDs. The recommendations that were outlined in Chapter 3 should be followed. Most donors are anonymous, but identified donors can be used if they go through the same rigorous screening and quarantine.

Husband insemination is commonly used to treat male factor infertility or infertility of unknown origin. It is also used if there is a cervical mucus disorder. Many times ovulation drugs are given to the female partner in concert with IUI.

Male disorders that are treated with IUI are malformations of the penis, retrograde ejaculation where the sperm goes into the bladder rather than outward, or impotence. IUI is also an option for males who have frozen their semen before a vasectomy or when facing cancer treatment.

The use of IUI for poor sperm parameters such as low counts or motility is open to debate. If there is a mild sperm problem, IUI may be quite useful. More severe forms of male infertility generally will not respond to IUI.

Furthermore, other parameters need to be optimal for this procedure to work even with mild male factor infertility. This procedure may not be ideal if the woman is older than 35 or if she has infertility problems that affect the pelvis such as moderate to severe endometriosis.

Lifestyle modifications outlined in Chapter 3 are important to IUI success. It is recommended that the woman undergo an evaluation before treatment with IUI. The best chance of success is within the first three to four cycles.

The semen used for a husband IUI is collected just before the procedure. Semen from a donor is thawed immediately prior to an insemination.

The day of insemination can be determined by several methods that predict when ovulation will occur. The first method is the use of LH urinary kits. An insemination is usually performed the day after the kit shows a positive result.

Another way would be to follow the patient with vaginal ultrasounds to assess follicle growth and then give a drug that triggers ovulation. This procedure is described in Chapter 5. The woman lies on the examination table, and a speculum and the insemination catheter are inserted. This procedure should take only a matter of minutes.

Azoospermia

Azoospermia refers to an absence of sperm in the ejaculate. This can be caused by one of two conditions:

1. Absence of sperm production (non-obstructive azoospermia).

2. Blockage of the ducts (obstructive azoospermia) that carry the sperm.

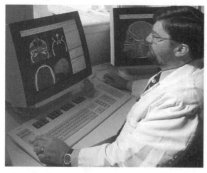

Non-obstructive azoospermia

NOA relates to a hormonal problem in the control mechanism in the brain – the hypothalamus or pituitary gland – or to a problem within the testicles.

These hormonal problems are not common. But some are correctable and must be investigated. Men with this condition usually have low blood levels of testosterone and low pituitary hormones FSH and LH. These men should have a blood-level check for prolactin and an MRI of the pituitary gland.

NOA is most commonly a direct testicular problem. Blood tests show a high FSH and a low or normal testosterone. This is the hormone that stimulates the production of sperm and it is high because the pituitary gland in the brain is trying to stimulate an increased production. In this disorder, the ejaculate volume is relatively normal and the ducts that carry the sperm out are normal. Sperm can be recovered from the testicles in 40 percent of these males. That sperm can subsequently be used for IVF.

A common cause of this problem is genetic, and therefore genetic testing is important. The problem lies on the Y chromosome. The Y chromosome has two parts – a short arm and a long arm. On the long arm of the Y chromosome, there is an area that is responsible for directing sperm production. There are three areas called AZFa, b, and c. If deletions occur here, sperm production is impaired. If there is a deletion in AZFa and/or b, then the chance of finding sperm within the testicle is almost zero. There is no point in trying to extract sperm. If the deletion occurs in AZFc, there could be sperm in the ejaculate or in the testicles.

This gene defect is found in 5 to 6 percent of men with very low sperm counts and more than 10 percent of men with no sperm. Extracting sperm from the testicle is worthwhile. It can be used for IVF. All these genetic mutations will be passed on to sons born by IVF. Other genetic mutations or a refinement of the concepts presented will occur.

The extraction technique is called TESE, for testicular sperm extraction. This is a surgical procedure for extraction of sperm from the testicles, and it requires anesthesia.

Another genetic problem associated with no sperm or extremely low sperm counts is called Klinefelter's syndrome, which is a condition associated with an extra X chromosome. The man is then XXY instead of the normal XY.

There are different manifestations of this disorder that range from lack of puberty to merely a sperm problem. The men who come to us with simply a no-sperm problem in the ejaculate may have sperm in the testicle. Therefore, TESE can be performed and the sperm used for IVF.

Obstructive azoospermia

Obstructive azoospermia implies that a duct that carries the sperm out is congenitally absent or obstructed. The most common cause of such an obstruction is a vasectomy.

Reversal of a vasectomy by microsurgical technique is very successful and allows a spontaneous pregnancy without risks of multiple births from fertility drugs. If the time from vasectomy to surgical reversal is too long – typically more than fifteen years – success rates drop. If there is a female infertility problem requiring IVF, this option may need to be reassessed.

The average interval from vasectomy reversal surgery to pregnancy is twelve to eighteen months. If reconstruction of the obstructed ducts is not possible, sperm needs to be extracted directly from the testicle and used for IVF.

Absence of the vas deferens – the duct that carries the sperm from the testicle outward – also can be congenital. Men with this condition have low semen volume as well as no sperm because many times the seminal vesicle that produces a substantial part of the semen is also absent. The congenital absence of the vas deferens is associated with congenital absence of the kidney in some patients.

A congenital bilateral absence of the vas deferens is called CBAVD. An experienced male infertility specialist easily makes this diagnosis through a physical examination.

Almost all men with cystic fibrosis have no sperm. That is the result of absence of the vas deferens. Both testicles are adversely affected. However, males can be born with CBAVD as the only manifestation of cystic fibrosis, and therefore testing is critical for both the man and his partner because either one can carry the gene. The treatment to get sperm is surgical; this surgical extraction of the sperm is called MESA (microsurgical epididymal sperm aspiration) or PESA (percutaneous epididymal sperm aspiration).

Cystic fibrosis is a disease that causes thick secretions to accumulate in the lung and the pancreas. It is most frequently found in Caucasians of Ashkenazi Jewish or European descent. However, CF can affect all ethnic groups. It is a genetic disorder with a mutation of the CF gene. CF is found if there are mutations on both copies of the CF gene. Mutations found on one copy result only in a carrier state.

However, if both partners of the couple have one copy of the mutation, their child can inherit the mutated copy from each parent and develop the disease, or that child may inherit the mutated copy from one parent only and simply be a carrier. In addition, the children can inherit the normal copy from each parent. This issue is complex and needs investigation and management.

For example, there are at least 1,000 different mutations, and tests will detect most but not all of them. The most common mutation is the "delta F508 gene," especially in Caucasians of northern European descent. The typical test for screening assesses twenty-three mutations. This is the test recommended as a screen. The extended panel is recommended in males with CBAVD. The males born with CBAVD and no other manifestation all have a mutation on both copies of the CF gene. It happens that the gene defect is such that it will only manifest itself as CBAVD. These mutations are sometimes referred to as 5 T abnormalities.

Front-line perspectives

Anthony J. Thomas, Jr., M.D., has been a male infertility specialist for more than twenty-five years. He is co-author of the book *Overcoming Male Infertility: Understanding Its Causes and Treatments* (John Wiley & Sons, Inc., 2000). Dr. Thomas analyzes male infertility factors, develops treatment plans, and often performs corrective surgery to address those factors. There are a number of male infertility specialists in this country and abroad who have been trained by Dr. Thomas.

"It's a matter of pride for most men. They are afraid – not afraid physically, but afraid of what they may have to do, and they're embarrassed. We are going into the most intimate parts of their lives and they come in and meet a perfect stranger. For example, they meet me for the first time and I tell them to go into a room, close the door, and produce a semen sample. That's not an easy assignment.

"If I had one message I could give men who are having infertility issues it would be 'Don't be ashamed.'

"If I had a second message it would be 'Don't feel guilty. It's not your fault.'

"So many of these men think, 'My wife wants children, I want children, and it's my fault we don't have any.' They've done absolutely nothing wrong. It's just a fact of life that they were born with a low sperm count or no sperm or that their sperm for some reason or another is not effective.

"They think, 'I'm not really a man unless I can produce children.' They equate sexuality with reproduction. That's what we need to get away from. You can have totally normal male hormones and sexuality and totally abnormal sperm-forming capacity. You can't have it the other way around. You can't have normal sperm-forming capacity with abnormal male hormones.

"Once patients know that, they can separate it. They can begin to see that even if they're not making sperm, they are for the most part normal, healthy men who just aren't making the sperm to do the fertilization job. These people aren't sick. They just have some issues. But they are scared. They're embarrassed.

"Men fear they'll find out something they don't want to know. They fear they'll find out they don't have sperm. They fear they'll find out I have to operate on them and they don't want that. Women handle these things better. If men had to bear children, there would be no population problem.

"Semen analysis is not like going for a urine analysis where you give a little bit of your urine and it's all the same in your bladder. Semen analysis is much different. Number one, you have to abstain from intercourse for a couple of days to get a full sample. You have to have some sort of maximum stimulation to give a really good sample. You have to be relaxed and know you are going to give a sample, so take your time. This is not self-pleasuring. This is hard work.

"We give them a room with a bed and a sink and a bathroom where they can wash their hands so they don't feel they're being shoved in a closet to do some 'dirty' thing. We make it as clean and neat and comfortable as possible. What we're asking them to do is important. They're not going in there to enjoy this. They're going in there because they have to go in there. They have to do this. We don't ever want them to think we're asking them to do something dirty.

"Patients are smart, but they are often misguided. They have gone on the Internet and Googled infertility. You can find so many references you won't be done for a year and you may never hit the same page twice. There's a lot of good stuff on the Internet, but you have to be selective.

"My message for couples is to approach this as a couple's problem. Be serious about it. But don't lose your sense of humor. Sometimes, take a break. If you are a prayerful person, then pray. You are working with the person you love to achieve a common goal and you both have to have the same degree of desire to achieve this. For women, they have a reminder they are not pregnant every single month. They get very depressed. They cry. They get very emotional. Guys need to understand this.

"Most of our male patients do not need drugs. Only a small number have a hormone deficiency or have had cancer radiation or chemotherapy treatments in the past or an infection now that would require some sort of drug therapy.

"It is also a fact that some men have conditions that cannot be corrected surgically. An example of that would be a man who was born without a vas deferens, which is an essential part of the male reproductive system that cannot be created surgically. In those cases, we may do a sperm aspiration procedure or biopsy the testicles to find sperm to freeze now and save for later in vitro fertilization.

"More often than not, however, we find ourselves dealing with one form of blockage or another and those conditions are addressed with microsurgery.

"Our experience tells us that you can never completely rule out male factor infertility. Short of zero sperm, there can always be some male factor along the way. So we continue to work with the couple. That is why ongoing communication between the woman's gynecologist and the man's urologist is so important. It's essential for those communication lines to remain open.

"Sometimes we really don't do anything for anybody except become their cheerleader. I got a letter from a man who said another hospital told him to look for donor sperm. He came to me and I told him I thought he had enough sperm to get this done. That's all I did. But he said giving him confidence was very important. He sent me a picture of his twins.

"I had another case where the people drove hundreds of miles to show me their baby. They were just so happy they wanted to do this."

Karen Seifarth is on the front line with the Cleveland Clinic Andrology Laboratory and Sperm Bank. She and her associates work with a variety of male infertility issues that lead to insemination. They also are responsible for cryopreservation of sperm, which can be a key strategy for patients where generating sperm regularly is a problem or they need to freeze sperm in advance of chemotherapy or radiation treatments.

She says, "After the first time, guys get comfortable with the fact that it's simply a masturbation-collected sample. Once they get over the fact that they know that we know what they're doing, they're generally okay. I tell them to forget about us. We have work to do. We have other things going on. For us, it's just another sample.

"We have patients come to us from our cancer center. These are young men recently diagnosed with cancer for which they will undergo either chemotherapy or radiation. Those treatments can affect fertility in the future. So we freeze

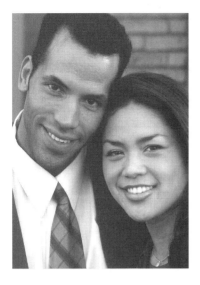

their sperm. All of our sperm depositors sign a contract that says if they die before the sperm is used, no rights to that frozen sperm transfer to any other family member unless there is a court order. We take no word of mouth. We require a death certificate.

"We also see a lot of couples trying to conceive through artificial insemination. Their stress levels are very high. This can drive a couple apart. Couples need to talk about their issues.

"We see some couples who are so loving that we know that even if they can't conceive, they will still be married in the future."

Frequently asked questions

Q. How quickly can you tell me if I have a problem?

A. We can tell there is a problem with just one semen analysis. However, it takes time to figure out exactly what the problem is and what treatment can be offered.

Q. I'm really mortified by what you may ask me to do. Who can I talk about this with so I can get over the embarrassment factor?

A. Patients can speak to their doctor or any member of the infertility team about any issue they feel they need to discuss. These professionals have experience talking about any issue.

Q. Is it normal to feel awkward about discussing these issues with my wife?

A. Issues of sexuality and fertility can be difficult topics for couples. However, it is important to work these issues out so as to achieve some harmony in the treatment objectives. Professional counseling may be necessary.

Q. Do I have to miss much work to get the tests you recommend?

A. The tests for men are more limited than for women. However, if an abnormality is found, several appointments may be necessary to investigate and treat the problem. In addition, men often choose to be with their wives for many of their procedures.

Q. What's the best thing I can do to support my wife as she goes through her part of this?

A. Communication and sensitivity are the two most important support mechanisms to offer your spouse.

Q. What should I expect in the way of support from her?

A. Hopefully, the same things she expects from you – good communication and sensitivity.

Q. I am shocked to hear that so much of the infertility issue is related to men. Does the experience of your practice really support that?

A. It comes as a surprise because men usually equate sexuality with fertility. Many men believe that if their sex life is fine, fertility should not be an issue. Thus, they are often surprised when we do find a male infertility problem. The facts speak for themselves – many men have an infertility issue.

Q. What would be the normal recovery period for some of the different micro-surgeries?

A. That depends on the surgery. For example, a vasectomy reversal may be a few days to return to sedentary work and three weeks to full physical activity, including sexual activity. A varicocele, on the other hand, may take a week in terms of a normal recovery.

Q. Is there any potential risk to male sexuality from microsurgical procedures?

A. We want you to understand that sexuality and fertility are separate. Therefore, risks of surgery to address infertility are related to that issue, not your sexuality.

Q. If a man (or a woman) has a history of a sexually transmitted disease, how much risk does that STD pose with respect to being able to conceive? How much risk to a baby?

A. In women, an STD is clearly associated with infertility. In men, it is not as clear. The risk to the baby is dependent on the type of STD. For example, a previous chlamydia infection poses no risk. On the other hand, previous HIV or hepatitis B infection poses significant risk to a baby.

Q. What's the rate of success for vasectomy reversals?

A. That depends on the interval of time between the vasectomy and the reversal. It also depends on the technique of the vasectomy and, of course, on the skill of the surgeon who performs the reversal. As we have already discussed, pregnancy rates also depend on the age and fertility status of the woman. If all conditions are ideal, success rates for a vasectomy reversal are among the highest for any infertility procedure.

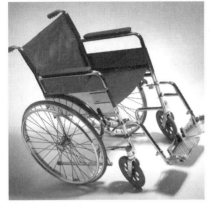

Patient talk

Sherri and Steve were married several years and had begun to think about having a family. They were just waiting to be in a little stronger financial position.

"We had all these dreams," Sherri says. "In a matter of one moment, everything changed."

Steve was 34 years old. Sherri was 25 when the type of accident that you always think will happen only to "other people" happened to Steve. Employed by a landscaping company, he was trimming a tree. He fell. He nearly died. Now, he spends his days in a wheelchair paralyzed from the waist down.

His body was broken, but his spirit was not. And neither was Sherri's.

"We decided we wanted to continue with our lives as normally as possible, including having children," Steve says. "I asked my spinal cord specialist if I would still be able to father children. He said yes. We learned the choices would be either artificial insemination or in vitro fertilization.

"My sister knew someone who had been to the Cleveland Clinic for infertility treatments. We went there. They retrieved a sperm specimen from me to determine motility. I was okay on that issue, but one of the results of my injury was that I could no longer ejaculate. The only way this was going to work was for the doctor to do a procedure to take some of my sperm and freeze it for use later.

"Based on my situation, we had to choose between the far less expensive artificial insemination option or the far more successful, but much more costly IVF. We went right to IVF."

Steve and Sherri used a procedure called IVF-ICSI, in which a single sperm is injected directly into an egg in vitro, with the resulting embryo placed back in the uterus. Steve's sperm was frozen while they waited for the optimum time for the procedure. Eventually, two embryos were implanted. The result? Twin boys.

But before they could do that, they also had to deal with an issue of Sherri's – ovarian cysts, which were removed surgically. This is a good example of a case where both partners had issues.

Steve says, "The hardest thing we had to do was to prepare ourselves if we were not successful. We were lucky. We hit on the first cycle. But if that hadn't happened, we wouldn't have stopped until we ran out of money.

"The worst advice we got was from people who kept asking if we were going to spend all our money when Sherri might not get pregnant. A lot of people said that. But the best advice came from people who said the odds were in our favor. I kept thinking of that when I started to worry."

"Being able to have these two little guys with Steve being hurt really brought our dreams back. This is proof that anything is possible," Sherri says.

From his wheelchair, Steve looks you directly in the eye and adds, "These guys are little miracles.

"My message is don't give up. Do your homework. Learn as much as you can about the different medical facilities and options you have. That's not as difficult as people think. You don't have to remember all the different medical terms, just the concepts."

He adds, "We are blessed."

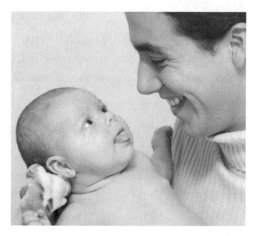

Summary

Men need to get on board in terms of being "in the program." Infertility belongs to both of you – not just the other person in your house.

If you really want to get into the best medical hands, get affiliated with a practice that includes a male infertility urology specialist. That is such a potential advantage in terms of integrated treatment plans as well as enhanced patient communication.

We started this book with the theme "You're Not Alone." Gentlemen, that applies to you as well as to your partner. You are not the first and you most certainly will not be the last man to require some sort of procedure. And just as your partner needs you to lean on, you will not be alone if you have a supportive spouse.

Chapter 7
In Vitro Fertilization

By the time you are ready to go forward with in vitro fertilization, you already will have gone through these four steps at a minimum:

1. You will have selected an infertility specialist.

2. You and your partner will have experienced a series of medical tests.

3. You both will have taken whatever medical steps are necessary to address your infertility issues.

4. You will have reached agreement with your infertility specialist that your best chance to become pregnant is with IVF.

When in vitro fertilization was first introduced in the late 1970s, it was hailed as a breakthrough. Many couples who had never been able to achieve pregnancy were able to have babies thanks to IVF.

Over time, it has become increasingly effective. Today, more children are being conceived with fewer embryos on average than ever before.

For almost thirty years, IVF continues to represent a breakthrough for infertility treatment. "Miracle babies" are born every day thanks to ever-evolving IVF technology.

But as our institution points out in its informational materials, there have also been other breakthroughs since the development and introduction of IVF.

In the 1980s, these included embryo freezing, transvaginal ultrasonography, and operative laparoscopy.

And in the 1990s, two other breakthroughs occurred. One was pre-implantation genetic testing and the other was ICSI, which is short for intracytoplasmic sperm injection.

Intracytoplasmic sperm injection is a perfect example of a long and potentially very intimidating term that you do not need to remember. But the concept is very simple and well worth knowing about. You may want to remember these four letters – ICSI.

In traditional in vitro fertilization, multiple eggs and sperm in a laboratory environment are placed in a petri dish. If all goes well, an egg and a sperm unite and are placed back in the woman's uterus as an embryo.

IVF-ICSI is a first cousin of that approach and is accomplished in a laboratory, where a single sperm is injected directly into a single egg. This is described in further detail in the section that follows titled "Medically speaking."

ICSI is only one option beyond traditional IVF.

Plain talk

If there really was such a thing as an "average patient," there would be a step-by-step progression to IVF.

For example, you would probably try some drug therapy for a while. In addition, one or both of you might have some sort of surgical procedure to address one of the conditions described in this book. After that, you might have moved on to a series of inseminations. At this point, a year or more would likely have gone by.

If there were no results at the insemination level, you would likely then step up to in vitro fertilization. It is always risky to generalize, but with the caveat that there are exceptions, that pretty well describes a standard progression through infertility treatment.

One notable exception to this order would be a couple in which the woman's biological clock is really beginning to tick loudly. In that case, it is very likely we would recommend accelerating the process by going to IVF almost immediately after your medical evaluations.

Other exceptions might occur if the female pelvic disease is so severe or chances for a successful outcome with insemination are so low that IVF is the only choice that makes sense.

If you are in a position to make choices, you need to think very carefully. You want to do everything reasonable so you never, ever have to look back with any regrets. But in this scenario, the operative word is *reasonable*.

What is reasonable for one person may be entirely unreasonable for somebody else. Truly, it is in the eye of the beholder. Here, then, are some questions you may want to ask yourself and also discuss with your spouse.

- How willing am I to go through a continuum of increasingly complex procedures over what may be many months? Do I have the emotional strength to do this? Do I have the personal staying power to get through this?

- Would it be better to go with an easier and less costly but statistically less successful procedure first, such as insemination, or should I ratchet up immediately to the far more expensive IVF procedure, which has been shown to produce much better results?

- What are my financial resources and what is my risk tolerance with respect to those resources? If I fail at the lower-success-rate procedures, will I still have enough money left for a good shot at the more expensive IVF?

- If I go through with IVF, how many embryos will I want to have frozen? If I am successful at an early IVF attempt, what will I want to do with those extra embryos?

Those are extremely important questions. Throughout the process of addressing infertility issues, there is a constant requirement to manage your own expectations. And if there are two of you going through the process, it is also extremely important that you are in agreement with respect to these issues. So if you have choices, please do all you can to choose well.

Medically speaking

As you know, the technology that is used for assisted reproduction is called ART (assisted reproductive technology).

A center that offers ART has procedures that handle gametes (sperm and egg). This includes preparation of sperm for intrauterine insemination, preparation of eggs for fertilization, and freezing or transferring of gametes or embryos back into the body.

Fertilization of eggs can be achieved through a variety of techniques such as insemination (putting sperm around the eggs) or direct injection of the sperm into an egg. As stated earlier, direct injection of the sperm into the egg is called intracytoplasmic sperm injection (ICSI).

The ART laboratory manages embryos by preparing them for transfer into the uterus or by freezing them for further use.

The general concept that fertilization of an egg is occurring outside the body (in vitro) rather than inside the body (in vivo) is called in vitro fertilization. The first IVF baby was born in 1978. Since then, hundreds of thousands of babies have been born from these techniques.

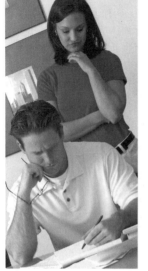

Pre-IVF discussion

Before starting an IVF cycle, there are several topics that need to be discussed with the IVF medical group.

First, there should be a reality-based discussion about your chance of success. This means a review of the center's reported statistics and how your own personal history will modify the outcome.

Ovarian reserve testing results should be reviewed because this will have an impact on the outcome. The details of ovarian reserve testing are covered in Chapter 4. Women with mildly elevated FSH levels still can proceed to IVF as long as it is understood that pregnancy rates will be lower.

The physician should review your medical record to determine whether anything can be done to improve your IVF outcome. This sometimes means performing a procedure that will not help to achieve a spontaneous pregnancy but will help with IVF. The best example of that is what is called a prophylactic salpingectomy. This means that damaged uterine tubes (fallopian tubes) are surgically removed pre-IVF. It is thought that the fluid in some damaged tubes (called hydrosalpinx) may have a negative effect on embryo implantation. The tubes usually are removed by laparoscopy. This procedure can be risky at times since there may be scar tissue around the tubes that involves the bowel.

The next step is to ensure that all the pre-IVF tests are done and are normal. This typically includes blood tests and cervical cultures for STDs. (Many blood tests for antibodies are suggested by some IVF centers. These tests are expensive. Credible studies have shown absolutely no value to them. The consensus is that they should not be performed.)

Good nutrition, stress management, and other parameters discussed in Chapter 3 should be followed. No alcohol, caffeine, or smoking is allowed. Excessive weight will diminish IVF outcome. Try to deal with these issues of smoke cessation or counseling before starting with IVF. Of course, stress management during the cycle is important, too.

An evaluation of the uterine cavity and cervix is necessary before IVF is started. The uterine cavity should be normal without any polyps or fibroids. If any abnormality is found in an area where it may affect the pregnancy rate, it should be removed. All fibroids and polyps larger than 5 mm are usually removed before proceeding.

Scar tissue (adhesions) within the cavity should be removed as well. Sometimes a congenital anomaly of the uterus, such as a uterine septum, is found. If there also is a problem with previous miscarriages, all agree that the septum should be removed before IVF. It is somewhat more controversial if the septum occurs without a history of recurrent miscarriages. However, most infertility specialists would remove a uterine septum.

The uterine cavity can be evaluated by different techniques. The first is by X-ray (hysterosalpingogram or HSG), in which contrast dye is injected into the uterine cavity. The advantage of this technique is that the uterine tubes can be assessed very effectively.

Another method to evaluate the uterine cavity is by ultrasound (saline infusion sonohysterogram or SIS). The advantage of this technique is that there are no X-rays and it is considered less painful than the HSG procedure. However, it is more difficult to assess the uterine tubes with the SIS.

Another technique to assess the uterine cavity is a hysteroscopy, which is performed in an office setting and involves inserting a small camera through the cervix into the uterus. A direct visual assessment of the cavity is obtained in this way.

These approaches are all similar in obtaining the desired information. A mild analgesic such as ibuprofen is required one hour before any of these procedures.

The next pre-IVF assessment procedure is the "mock" or trial embryo transfer. This, too, is done in an office setting. The level of difficulty, depth, and pathway required to introduce the embryo transfer catheter into the uterus is assessed during this evaluation. The information is recorded and made available to the doctor performing the transfer. If there are difficulties, perhaps something can be done beforehand such as dilation of the cervix.

A review of the semen analysis or any other potential procedures to obtain sperm should be discussed and arrangements made to have a urologist available if needed. Some centers recommend that sperm be frozen for use in case there are difficulties obtaining a fresh sample of acceptable quality. A drug such as sildenafil (Viagra) may need to be available to ensure the necessary sperm collection.

There are many questions that should be discussed before proceeding.

- How many doctors are on your team and what are the chances that your personal physician will be doing the IVF procedure?

- If necessary, will the embryologist be available to discuss outcomes?

- Ask the nurse member of the team to explain the stimulation protocol in detail.

- What are the limits on what a nurse can tell you?

- What drugs will be used?

- How often will you have monitoring to make sure everything is fine?

- Will an oral contraceptive be used first to decrease cyst formation and synchronize follicles?

- What happens if the ovaries will not stimulate?

- Will the cycle be canceled?

- What happens if you stimulate too much?

- Will you have enough medication to last over holidays or weekends?

It is very important to review the amount of medication required over weekends and holidays. It is quite expensive and you may not want to keep too much extra medication on hand. In that case, an estimate of the weekend/holiday requirements is helpful. Also, find out about the pharmacies that carry this type of medication.

Make a list of all phone numbers and key people you may need to call. For example, how do you get hold of the IVF team member on call or the embryology lab?

A clear understanding of the other procedures associated with IVF should be discussed.

- Will there be an ICSI procedure?

- Will PGD (preimplantation genetics) be recommended?

- What happens if there is no fertilization of the eggs?

- Will a rescue ICSI be performed?

- Do you want all eggs retrieved potentially fertilized? This implies creating more embryos than can be transferred back into the uterus at one time.

A decision needs to be made about the disposition of extra embryos. An immediate decision is usually easier. Most couples choose to freeze the extra embryos so that they can be used in case of failure of the current cycle or for future children if they are successful in the present cycle. Embryos are generally frozen (cryopreserved) on the third or fifth day after the retrieval. The far more difficult decision is what to do with the extra embryos after the number of desired children is achieved.

A decision on the number of embryos to replace is critical. This may change somewhat after the quality and quantity of the embryos obtained are known. The trend is to transfer fewer embryos. It would be uncommon to replace more than two embryos in a woman less than 35 years old.

In the event of a multiple gestation (triplets and higher), will you opt for what is referred to as selective reduction? If yes, that means that a procedure is performed under ultrasound guidance to decrease the number of embryos so that only one or two embryos are left. That is a huge decision. Think about it very, very carefully.

A discussion of the potential complications of IVF is important. The most common complication is multiple births. We consider this a complication because babies born from multiple births are at greater risk for prematurity and other pregnancy complications. Additional complications are discussed below.

Outcomes

In vitro fertilization offers very high success rates. These results come from dramatic improvements in clinical and laboratory techniques in recent years.

All clinics are required to report their IVF results to the Centers for Disease Control and Prevention. This information can be accessed through (http://www.cdc.gov/reproductivehealth/art.htm). We caution you that no direct comparisons should be made between clinics because the patient population can be different clinic to clinic.

The CDC reports state how many women these clinics have with diminished ovarian reserve, the diagnosis, and the type of ART that was performed. The outcomes are reported by age group (younger than 35, 35 to 37, 38 to 40, 41 to 42). The pregnancy rates will be presented by cycle-initiated retrieval and by embryo transfer. The average number of embryos transferred will be listed as well as the percent of pregnancies with multiple births (twins, triplets, and higher).

What is immediately apparent in the data is the substantial influence of age. Pregnancy rates drop dramatically after the age of 40 and are extremely uncommon after the age of 42. In patients age 43 and above, the pregnancy rate is 5.2

percent and the live birth rate is 2.0 percent. If you think your favorite celebrity is spontaneously pregnant at the age of 49, you may well be wrong. Most of those pregnancies are the result of donated eggs from younger women.

Miscarriages occur more frequently with increasing age. They occur to fewer than 13 percent of women under 35, but to more than 50 percent of women over 42. Most miscarriages are the result of chromosomal abnormalities.

Children born from ART

Today, there are an estimated 1.2 million children who have been born through in vitro fertilization since the first IVF baby more than two decades ago. One percent of newborns in the United States are now from ART.

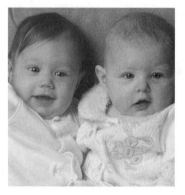

Assisted reproductive technology is responsible for the majority of multi-fetal pregnancies – twins, triplets, and higher born in the United States. These multi-fetal pregnancies are associated with significantly increased risk of adverse clinical outcome, including prematurity. The rate of neonatal mortality is four times as great among twins as it is for singletons. Morbidity such as cerebral palsy is increased in twins and especially in higher-level multiples.

Furthermore, the mother is at increased risk of adverse outcomes during pregnancy with multiples. Although most of the increased neonatal problems are attributed to multi-fetal gestations, even singletons may be at a slightly increased risk. Therefore, the obstetrician should always be aware that the baby was conceived from ART.

There is some recent evidence to suggest an increase in congenital anomalies (birth defects) among children born after in vitro fertilization or in vitro fertilization with ICSI or PGD. Keep in mind that congenital anomalies occur in 2 to 4 percent of newborn babies with mothers who were not treated for infertility. If there is a 30 percent increase in malformation rate, the rate after IVF would be between 2.6 percent and 5.2 percent. Although the data are somewhat controversial, overall there does not seem to be an increased risk of developmental problems in the children from ART, if we exclude those associated with multi-fetal births.

The process of IVF has several well-defined steps: ovarian stimulation, obtaining the egg and sperm, and transferring the embryo.

Ovarian stimulation protocols and monitoring

Most patients will be started on the ovarian stimulation protocol. This is a protocol in which a drug is given that shuts off the pituitary gland in the brain, which controls the ovaries. The pituitary gland is under control of the hypothalamus, which produces gonadotropin-releasing hormone (GnRH); GnRH controls FSH (follicle-stimulating hormone) and LH (luteinizing hormone) released from the pituitary gland. FSH and LH control the development of eggs and hormones (such as estrogen) from the ovary.

In the typical "long protocol," a drug that resembles GnRH (called an agonist) is used. In the U.S., leuprolide acetate or nafarelin are most commonly prescribed. These provide optimal control of the cycle to prevent premature ovulation and to maximize the number of eggs retrieved. The number of canceled IVF cycles resulting from failure to ovulate are fewer with the use of an agonist.

There are usually more eggs retrieved with this protocol than with others. The drugs can be started in the mid-luteal phase (halfway between ovulation and the next period) or on the first or second day of your period. Starting in the mid-luteal phase appears to more quickly suppress the pituitary gland. There also may be less ovarian cyst formation, which can occur when using these drugs.

The initial response of an agonist actually is to increase rather than decrease FSH and LH. This is called the "flare" effect and lasts approximately two days. Then suppression occurs.

Sometimes a hormone such as the birth-control pill is used for one menstrual cycle before starting with an agonist. Some studies have shown that use of a hormone may decrease the formation of cysts. Typically, the GnRH agonist (such as leuprolide) is started at a high dose for ten days or so and then the dose is cut in half. Suppression is presumed when some vaginal bleeding occurs and confirmed with a blood test and an ultrasound. This ultrasound and blood test are sometimes referred to as a "baseline" ultrasound. Suppression usually takes about ten days but may in fact take two to three weeks. Suppression implies a low estrogen (estradiol) level and no ovarian cysts. The presence of an ovarian cyst is not necessarily a contraindication to starting ovarian stimulation as long as your estrogen level is low.

Next, the ovaries need to be stimulated with a gonadotropin drug (FSH alone or in combination with LH). This actually stimulates the ovary to produce eggs. The dose is based on age, weight, ovarian reserve testing response, and previous stimulated cycles. Patients with polycystic ovary syndrome may be started on lower doses.

These drugs are given subcutaneously (injected under the skin). Then to assess how the drug is stimulating the ovary, an ultrasound and a blood test for estrogen are performed at a frequency determined by the individual response to the protocol. The ultrasound will show the developing follicles as well as endometrial thickness. It is important to understand that a follicle is visible on ultrasound, but an egg is not. A follicle has some dimensions when ready, while to see an egg requires a microscope. A follicle is essentially a group of cells surrounding a fluid-filled cavity with the egg placed in one area off-center. Microscopic cells called a cumulus surround the egg. Not all follicles will yield an egg when aspirated.

Usually after five days of stimulation, the level of estrogen should be adequate. Dosage levels are then usually adjusted downward. The monitoring and drugs are continued until there is at least one follicle of 18 mm and two others of 16 mm. This endpoint is variable, and these stated endpoints are considered an acceptable minimum. Typically, we would expect a large number of follicles over 18 mm.

If the initial response to this protocol is poor, such as developing fewer than five follicles, the dose of the gonadotropin can be raised. However, although many infertility programs try this approach, most studies have not shown it to be a major benefit in changing either the number of eggs retrieved or pregnancy rates.

When the follicles have reached the appropriate size, hCG is given subcutaneously to start the process of ovulation. This process allows the egg to complete a cell division it started when it was in the uterus. The egg is then floating in the fluid and is ready to be aspirated. Retrieval is scheduled thirty-four to thirty-eight hours after hCG administration.

The choice of the gonadotropin is somewhat controversial. Most centers use a synthetic version FSH drug. These are convenient to use now that they come in multi-dose formats, which allow great flexibility for fine-tuning the dose. They are not derived from human fluids, but are made synthetically. The main limitation is their expense and the lack of any LH. However, FSH is the main gonadotropin necessary for egg development.

The typical protocol that causes pituitary suppression still has enough LH circulating. That is to say, the suppressed pituitary still produces sufficient LH to allow the cycle to proceed. However, in extreme suppression such as when an oral contraceptive is used first, the pituitary may not produce any LH. In those cases, an LH-containing drug may be added.

Alternative protocols

A poor responder is defined as having retrieved four eggs or less from a previous cycle or having canceled the cycle because there were four follicles or less.

Poor responders from previous cycles or anticipated poor responders for future cycles can be started on several different protocols. Low estrogen levels can also be seen as a poor responder. These patients can be tried on alternative regimens.

These alternative regimens will differ from center to center in terms of specific details. Most regimens start with higher doses of gonadotropins.

One approach is to decrease the dose and length of time of the GnRH agonist drug. In this protocol, called the microdose leuprolide protocol, the oral contraceptive is usually given for about one month and then stopped. It is thought that the use of the oral contraceptive may synchronize the available pool of follicles. A period will ensue and a smaller dose of GnRH agonist is given on the first day of the period or five days after the last oral contraceptive pill. The next day, a gonadotropin is started. The monitoring occurs the same way as the long protocol and both drugs are continued to the day of hCG. Since no suppression is required, the time to retrieval is far shorter.

Another approach, called the flare protocol, starts the GnRH agonist the day before the gonadotropin, and the drugs are given daily. In this way, there is no initial suppression of the ovaries as there is with the long protocol.

Yet another approach is to start the same way as the long protocol but stop the agonist earlier than the day of the hCG. The drug is stopped when the gonadotropins are started or early on in the stimulation.

A newer idea is to use a GnRH antagonist instead of an agonist. An antagonist suppresses the cycle within one day compared to the agonist, which usually takes more than a week. There is no flare effect, the initial temporary increase seen with an agonist. In this protocol, an oral contraceptive is given similar to the minidose agonist protocol. The gonadotropin is started five days after the last pill or when the period starts. An antagonist such as cetrorelix or ganirelix is started when the largest follicle reaches the right size.

These drugs are given subcutaneously. The cycle is monitored, as the other protocols are, with ultrasound and blood tests. The dose is sometimes adjusted up or down on day six of stimulation. Usually when the follicle reaches approximately 14 mm, a gonadotropin that also contains LH is added. This is important because the suppression of the pituitary is felt to be so profound that some LH should be added back.

None of these protocols seems superior, but the trend is to use either the mini-dose agonist protocol or the antagonist protocol.

You certainly do not need to understand or retain the technical terms. What you do need to remember is that there are options and that an experienced infertility specialist and practice can look at all of the options appropriate to your individual circumstances.

Retrieving eggs

Antibiotics are given at the time of egg retrieval to decrease the potential risk of infection from the procedure. Antibiotics are continued orally to decrease potential for transferring bacteria into the uterine cavity at the time of embryo transfer.

The retrieval procedure is performed under "conscious sedation." The level of sedation depends on the patient and the infertility center. Most centers give some narcotic intravenously, such as fentanyl, and a sedative that is typically similar to diazepam, such as midazolam. Some centers perform a local anesthetic block. Others will give a deeper form of sedation and sometimes even an epidural. The sedation level depends on the patient. Obesity makes the choice of sedation more complex.

A needle is passed into the follicle through a guide attached to an ultrasound probe. The fluid is quickly aspirated and given to embryologists who will immediately look for an egg. If there is no egg in the follicle, the follicle is sometimes "flushed" to see whether an egg can be detached. Most but not all follicles will contain an egg. It is uncommon when there are no eggs obtained from any of the follicles. When that happens, it is often due to an error in administering the hCG or other problem with the drug.

After the procedure, the patient stays in the recovery area for one or two hours and then can be discharged. Usually just some acetaminophen is prescribed for pain. There may be some minor vaginal bleeding. Luteal phase progesterone support is started the next day.

Obtaining sperm

Sperm is usually obtained on the same day as the egg procedure. If a fresh specimen is not obtainable because of stress or unavailability of the partner, a previously frozen specimen can be thawed.

Sometimes there is no sperm in the ejaculate and it must be obtained through a surgical procedure.

The embryology lab

When the embryology lab gets both the sperm and the egg, it is then the responsibility of that lab to optimize the conditions to obtain an embryo that will result in a pregnancy. This mission requires a laboratory that has both the right personnel and quality control mechanisms. All embryology labs should be certified by the appropriate national agency.

When the follicle fluid is handed to the embryologist, the embryologist identifies what is known as the "egg complex." This complex contains the egg and the surrounding cells. The maturity of the egg is then assessed by the embryologist. The designation of a mature egg is called Metaphase II.

The egg is then readied for fertilization. After the sperm has been collected or a specimen thawed, the sample is prepared for insemination or injection.

Either of those procedures is performed several hours after collection of eggs.

Insemination is performed by placing sperm around the egg. The sperm has to go through the cells around the egg (called the cumulus mass). Then the sperm undergoes a change called the acrosome reaction. Next it binds to the shell surrounding the egg. The sperm then must penetrate this shell by releasing enzymes. After penetration of the shell, the sperm binds to the egg cell membrane. The genetic material in the sperm is then brought into the cell. To say the least, a lot of things have to go right.

In cases of male factor infertility, the egg will not fertilize with simple insemination and the sperm will be directly injected into the egg by ICSI. The cells around the egg are stripped off and the sperm is picked up by a micropipet and injected. The eggs are checked for fertilization the next morning.

If fertilization has occurred, the egg takes on a distinctive appearance. This results from two pronuclei that represent the male and female genetic material. The first day after fertilization is called the pronuclear stage, and the number and size of the pronuclei – which represent the male and female genetic material – are assessed. This one-cell stage is called a zygote. There are several other criteria used to assess the quality of fertilization. Typically, a member of the IVF team calls the couple at this time to report how many eggs have been fertilized.

The next day the embryo is assessed for cell number and appearance (morphology). The embryo is then assessed each day.

At seventy-two hours after retrieval, the embryo is called a "cleaved embryo." Typically, embryos are grown for transfer to either day three (cleaved embryo) or day five (called a blastocyst). The decision to transfer on day three or five remains a matter of debate in the medical community. Day five offers the advantage of selecting better embryos so as to transfer fewer. However, the disadvantage is that some good-quality embryos available on day three do not make it to the blastocyst stage.

On the day of the embryo transfer, a discussion with the embryologist or a member of the IVF team should take place about the quality of the embryos to be transferred. On day three (seventy-two hours after retrieval), the quality of the embryos is assessed by at least the following two general criteria:

1. The percent of fragmentation seen in the embryo.

2. The number and symmetry of the cells that are seen.

Fragmentation refers to production of cytoplasmic blebs (bubbles) within the embryo. The cause of these blebs is still unknown. The number of cells (called blastomeres) is usually two to four at the forty-eight-hour evaluation and six to eight at the seventy-two-hour evaluation. This is important to determine because, as previously stated, these are the criteria used to determine the quality of the embryos.

The cell quality is also assessed. Typically, these cells are relatively symmetrical. Ideally, there should be fewer than 20 percent fragments on day three after fertilization. Although there is a trend toward higher pregnancy rates with less fragmentation, pregnancies still occur even with a higher percentage of fragmentation.

Many other criteria are used to assess the embryo, but these are the most universally used.

Blastocysts have a characteristic shape that reflects the health of the embryo. A blastocyst has a cavity that is lined with cells. The embryologist looks to see whether the cavity is present and whether the cells that surround the cavity are normal in appearance.

The lab may perform some other procedures to optimize the ability of the embryo to implant and evolve into a viable pregnancy. These include assisted hatching and co-culture. The embryo must "come out of its shell" to implant properly. This process is referred to as hatching. Some embryos cannot hatch on their own because the shell is too hard or for some other unknown reason. "Assisted hatching" or "zona drilling" is performed to facilitate this process. It is done routinely in many embryology labs. In other labs this procedure is done selectively such as with patients of older reproductive age or IVF failure. The procedure can be done with an acidified solution or with a laser.

Co-culture is a technique that grows the embryos in the presence of other cell types. These cells are thought to help the embryo develop, although the mechanism is unclear.

Embryo transfer and luteal phase support

With IVF, embryo transfer is usually easy and without problems.

Typically, embryos are transferred back into the uterus on day three (cleaved embryo) or day five (blastocyst) after egg retrieval. Most embryo transfers are performed with ultrasound guidance. The uterine cavity appears like a triangle with the base at the top of the screen. The embryos are placed within this triangle.

Each person is different. Fluid is taken orally in appropriate quantities to fill the bladder. The sensation of a full bladder may not necessarily reflect an adequately filled bladder for embryo transfer.

A transabdominal probe is placed on the lower abdomen and the uterus identified. A speculum of appropriate size is then inserted and the mucus on the cervix is washed off. Usually the first pass is performed with a catheter without any embryos. The catheter is visualized during the insertion. The doctor already has the report of the trial embryo transfer.

If all goes well, embryos are then loaded in another catheter and transfer occurs. When the embryos are released, there is a distinct flash seen on ultrasound that persists after the catheter is withdrawn. The catheter is then checked to make sure there are no retained embryos. A rest period of thirty to sixty minutes is generally offered, although there are no data that show this makes a difference. Similarly, decreased activity and no hot tubs are generally recommended until the pregnancy test. But again, there are no data to support this recommendation. It just makes good sense.

There are certainly difficult embryo transfers that require patience and skill. Fortunately, most such transfers are anticipated beforehand so that everyone is ready. Several methods may help such as using a more rigid catheter or one that has an inner stylet, which is a rigid interior guide. Sometimes a tenaculum, a grasping forceps used on the cervix, is necessary.

The luteal phase (the time interval after ovulation) needs hormonal support. Both estrogen and progesterone are used to provide that support. The options for progesterone are intramuscular progesterone, vaginal progesterone, and subcutaneous hCG.

Vaginal progesterone can be formulated by a local pharmacy as a suppository. Many pills designed for oral use can be placed in the vagina and absorbed easily. Numerous studies have reported the effectiveness of this approach. A vaginal progesterone gel is approved for infertility and administered daily or twice per day. There is some variability on when the drug is initiated. Some programs start on the same day of the egg retrieval while others start on the next day.

Drugs are continued until pregnancy is confirmed. At that time, if injectable hormone support was used, it may be switched to a vaginal preparation and continued for at least thirty days. These protocols for luteal phase support are similar regardless of the ovarian stimulation protocol.

Complications of IVF

There are several important potential complications of IVF to discuss:

- Risks of multiple birth.

- Possibility of ectopic pregnancy (a pregnancy that occurs outside the cavity of the uterus).

- Bleeding from the egg retrieval procedure or rupture of an ovarian cyst.

- Infection.

- Ovarian hyperstimulation syndrome (OHSS).

Bleeding can be severe to the extent that it requires transfusion or even surgery with loss of an ovary. Infection can be severe enough to require hospital admission with intravenous antibiotics and potentially even surgery with loss of pelvic organs. Fortunately, the extremes of these complications from IVF are uncommon.

There seems to be a consensus that no clear association exists between the use of IVF-related drugs and ovarian cancer.

Ectopic pregnancy may occur even if we put the embryos in the uterine cavity because they may float into the tube. Usually, they are transported back into the uterus by the tubes. However, if there is tubal disease, that may not happen.

Ovarian hyperstimulation syndrome

All patients have enlarged ovaries with IVF. However, it is far more dramatic in OHSS, in which fluid leaks from the vascular system into the abdomen.

The leaking of fluid from the vascular system causes blood changes, including concentration of red blood cells (hemoconcentration). The symptoms of this syndrome include abdominal discomfort, nausea, vomiting, and diarrhea. Worrisome symptoms are rapid weight gain, increasing abdominal girth, shortness of breath, and decreased urine output.

The syndrome typically starts three to seven days after administration of the hCG that triggers ovulation. A late form can occur two weeks after hCG triggers ovulation and is usually found in patients who are pregnant.

Women at risk for this syndrome include those with high estrogen concentrations on the day of hCG administration. This may include induced ovulation (retrieval of more than twenty eggs), a diagnosis of polycystic ovary syndrome, young age, low body weight, or a previous history of OHSS. Risk also increases with use of hCG support in the luteal phase. However, OHSS can occur even without these known risk factors. Pregnancy can increase the severity of the disease.

There are several proposed approaches to preventing this syndrome. Obviously, the only way to completely avoid OHSS is to avoid ovarian stimulation per se. This can be accomplished with a natural cycle IVF or in vitro maturation or both. In vitro maturation, a relatively new concept, will be discussed further in a section that follows.

If ovarian stimulation is likely to occur, other methods may be tried in high-risk patients.

The first is to replace or lower the dose of the hCG used to trigger ovulation. A GnRH agonist can be used to trigger ovulation. However, cases of OHSS have been reported after doing this. This drug cannot be used to induce ovulation if the ovarian stimulation encompassed what is called the long "down-regulation" protocol. In patients at risk for OHSS, luteal phase support is usually performed with progesterone rather than hCG.

Another way is to "coast" the cycle. This means that ovarian stimulation drugs are withheld until the estrogen level becomes acceptable. However, the wait may be so long (more than three days) that few viable eggs can be obtained. Furthermore, OHSS still can occur.

Yet another option is to freeze all the embryos. OHSS will have a less severe form if your infertility clinic does that. Since OHSS usually occurs between days three and seven, embryo transfer can be delayed until day five (blastocyst transfer) so that a further evaluation can be made in patients considered at risk.

There are some infertility specialists who recommend the administration of a blood product (such as albumin) at the time of egg retrieval. Although this is safe, there are risks of allergic reaction and the potential transmission of a virus.

If the syndrome occurs, its management requires careful monitoring. The patient should be vigilant about any symptoms, such as respiratory problems, that reflect a worsening situation. Sexual intercourse should be avoided. Analgesics and possibly anti-nausea medication may be required. The patient should drink at least one liter of an electrolyte-balanced drink (such as a sport drink) per day. Daily weight gain should be recorded and if it's more than two pounds, that should be reported to the IVF team immediately.

Communication with the team is required if the patient is at home. Although not confined to bed, a patient should not participate in any strenuous activity. If there are worsening symptoms, she should be re-evaluated and blood tests ordered.

Hospitalization may be required if that occurs. During hospitalization, the fluid intake and output will be closely monitored, weight measured, and ultrasound exams will be performed to assess the fluid in the abdomen. Sometimes it is necessary to drain the fluid in the abdomen with an ultrasound-guided needle aspiration.

The worst complication of this syndrome is related to blood-clotting events. Strokes have been reported. Therefore, an anticoagulant such as heparin may be prescribed. Ruptured cysts or torsion of an ovary requiring surgery is uncommon but possible.

Alternatives to traditional IVF

Gamete intrafallopian transfer (GIFT) transfers the egg and sperm into the uterine tube without fertilization. Fertilization should occur naturally in the tube.

The fertilized egg is called a zygote. Transfer of a zygote is called ZIFT (zygote intrafallopian transfer).

A cleaved embryo also can be transferred into the tube. It is called tubal embryo transfer (TET). The main disadvantage to this procedure is that it requires general anesthesia and laparoscopy to access the tube. Manipulating enlarged hyperstimulated ovaries to place the egg and sperm, the fertilized egg, or the embryo into the uterine tubes can be challenging. This substantially increases both the risks and costs. Furthermore, pregnancy rates are not higher. Nevertheless, this technique may be useful for patients who have an extremely difficult uterine transfer.

In vitro maturation

The ideal way to achieve IVF would be to avoid all ovulation induction drugs.

With in vitro maturation (IVM), eggs are retrieved by ultrasound as with standard IVF and these immature eggs are "matured" in the laboratory by special culture media. When they are mature, they are fertilized and the embryos transferred in the usual way.

IVM is available in a limited number of infertility centers at this time, but is promising for the future. IVM is especially useful in patients for whom ovarian stimulation with drugs is not possible because of time constraints (such as with cancer patients or if the response to medication is excessive as with polycystic ovary syndrome).

Cryopreservation

Sperm and egg tissue (ovarian or testicular) and embryos can be frozen (cryo-preserved). Pregnancy rates with the use of frozen sperm or embryos are very good. So far, freezing unfertilized eggs has been less successful. However, there has been improvement in this technology, and pregnancies have been reported from specialized infertility centers.

The potential use for freezing unfertilized eggs is both ethical and practical. Some patients do not want to create more embryos than will be transferred into the uterus. Therefore, extra eggs can be frozen and fertilized only when thawed. Some cancer patients who are at risk for egg damage from chemotherapy may choose to undergo IVF. However, if there is no partner, the extracted eggs can be frozen.

Sperm freezing is a relatively simple process. Cryopreserving normal sperm as a pre-vasectomy procedure offers good pregnancy rates when thawed and used for insemination. Cryopreservation of sperm from cancer patients also is possible and quite successful. However, because the quality of the thawed sperm may not be optimal, a procedure such as IVF and ICSI may be required.

Embryo cryopreservation has been available since at least 1983 when the first pregnancy was reported from a frozen thawed embryo. The technique is now universally available, and most infertility clinics are very successful at offering this service.

The pregnancy rates from a frozen-thawed cycle are also reported to national organizations and can be seen at the same CDC website discussed earlier – www.cdc.gov. Pregnancy rates are dependent on the age of the women at the time the fresh embryos were obtained. Pregnancy rates generally are about half the fresh cycle rates. Embryos that have been micro-manipulated with the ICSI or PGD processes also can be frozen successfully.

Embryos are able to be frozen at any stage of their development. Most infertility centers report freezing at the pronuclear stage, cleaved embryo stage, or blastocyst stage. The earlier pronuclear freezing has a higher survival rate, but this limits the number of embryos available to choose from for the fresh cycle embryo transfer that occurs on day three or five. So this option may be acceptable for patients who have a very large number of embryos. Freezing also can occur on day three post-fertilization.

Usually the best are chosen for transfer and if there are excellent-quality extra embryos, they also can be frozen the same day. Alternatively, the extra embryos can be left in culture and if they make it to blastocyst stage, they can be frozen. If the transfer will occur on day five, the extra blastocysts that are not transferred can be frozen.

The transfer of frozen thawed embryos can occur on a spontaneous ovulatory cycle or an artificial one. In a spontaneous cycle, a conventional ovulation process with a normal luteal phase needs to be documented. This does not guarantee that, on a subsequent cycle when the embryos will be transferred, it will be normal as well.

Artificial cycles can be induced in women with spontaneous cycles or in women without any cycle at all. Most IVF programs use artificial cycles. A typical artificial cycle starts with an oral estrogen drug on day one of the cycle, and the dose is then increased. The endometrium is then assessed by ultrasound for proper thickness.

Different standards exist as to what is "proper." If the endometrial thickness is acceptable, progesterone is started. The progesterone can be intramuscular (progesterone in oil) or intravaginal (micronized progesterone or gels). Examples of when embryos may be transferred are:

- After three days of progesterone if the embryo was frozen at the pronuclear or day two cleaved stage.

- After four days of progesterone if the embryo was frozen at the day three cleaved stage.

- After five or six days of progesterone if the embryo was frozen at the blastocyst stage.

Estrogen and progesterone are continued until ten to twelve weeks of pregnancy. Intramuscular progesterone is exchanged for a vaginal one after pregnancy has been confirmed.

If there is insufficient thickening of the endometrium, the dose can be increased and perhaps an alternative route selected. For example, the transdermal route (a patch) can be chosen or additional estrogen can be administered intra-vaginally.

Freezing ovarian or testicular tissue

Freezing testicular tissue is important for an IVF program. In this way, sperm can be obtained at a separate time than during an IVF cycle.

If the sperm procurement procedure occurs on the day of the egg retrieval and no sperm are found, the woman has gone through the entire process for nothing. Also, if no sperm are found, the couple must then explore other possibilities. Testicular tissue freezing offers the possibility of assessing the situation at a separate time and initiating an IVF cycle only if sperm are found.

Freezing sperm found at the time of a vasectomy reversal is also advantageous. If the vasectomy reversal surgery fails and IVF is necessary, frozen sperm are available.

Ovarian tissue cryopreservation is presently an experimental procedure that is offered to cancer patients. If a woman undergoes chemotherapy, she is at risk for ovarian damage. There are several options. One is to freeze ovarian tissue. This tissue can be obtained by laparoscopy, and small pieces of tissue can be frozen. The process effectively destroys all of the growing follicles, but the resting follicles (called primordial follicles) will survive. These can be transplanted back into the patient. However, this tissue can die quickly because there is no blood supply. Few pregnancies have been reported with this procedure. Furthermore, a clear evaluation of the cancer type is important because transplanting the ovarian tissue back in again may bring a return of the cancer.

Front-line perspectives

Nina Desai, Ph.D., is a board-certified embryologist who runs the IVF laboratory for the Cleveland Clinic. In simple terms, she and her team are the glue that bind a sperm with an egg in a laboratory environment. The embryo that results from this process is then put back into the woman's uterus to develop into a fetus and ultimately a baby.

"When I started with our IVF program in the early to mid-1990s, the IVF success rates were less than half of what they are today. And those lower rates were being achieved despite the fact that four or five embryos were routinely being put back with the objective of achieving just a single pregnancy.

"Our goal has been to reduce the number of embryos and still get good results. We have been able to do that even though we have essentially been putting back one less embryo than just a few years ago. Today, we are getting far better results and normally we now only put back two embryos in patients who are under the age of 39.

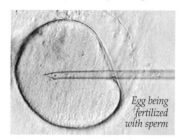

Egg being fertilized with sperm

"I tell people to go to the Centers for Disease Control website and look at clinics that are doing large volumes – over 100 IVF cycles at a minimum. Those are the ones with the most experience. There are some smaller programs that do well, but the larger the program the more resources available to patients and the more high-tech they are. Look at the age group results. With us, for example, the success rate is much higher for young women and much lower for the older patients. That is very typical and needs to be well understood. You can't generalize success.

"We have a research laboratory intimately associated with our IVF program. This means that when something new comes along, we perfect it in the lab and it's ready to go over to the clinical side much sooner.

"An example of that was a revolutionary new technique for freezing embryos. It was very exciting to us and looked like it would be great for clinical applications. Right away, we got one of our embryologists interested in doing some research on this technique. We worked out all the bugs. We became convinced that mouse embryos definitely looked better when frozen by this technique. We then went into a five-month clinical trial trying this new method on human embryos. We found that, yes, we were getting pregnancies, things looked just as good as our old protocol, and there was a better embryo survival rate. So now all of our patients are able to take advantage of this development. We followed exactly the same process when we implemented a procedure called pre-implantation genetic diagnosis.

"Today, most of our patients in the under-35 age group are producing thirteen to fourteen eggs and we are transferring on average approximately two embryos back to those women. If the other embryos look good, they are frozen for future use. But we always tell patients the pregnancy rate for frozen embryos is half that for fresh ones. Your best opportunity is with fresh embryos.

"We see some of the most severe cases of male factor infertility you can imagine. We might have three embryologists working six or seven hours just to find enough sperm to inject. Our lab can work wonders if the sperm has motility. But you have to have motility.

"People go on the Internet and think that everything that is published is true. People are more aware than they used to be, but in some ways there are lots of misconceptions because of what gets translated into short news bites. There are lots of celebrity pregnancies that are with donors. People don't understand that. It doesn't get reported. They don't understand the huge, huge impact of age. They feel young. They feel normal. They ask, how can my eggs be bad? They just don't understand.

"Ten years from now, I would speculate we will be using fewer drugs, putting back one embryo, and achieving pregnancy rates of 60 to 70 percent."

Frequently asked questions

Q. If I have a choice, isn't it really smart for me to go right to IVF?

A. This is a personal decision. Typically, we try to use the least interventional technique we can to achieve a pregnancy. However, some patients want the highest success rate procedures immediately.

Q. What if my spouse and I are not on the same page – should I stay in the program?

A. This program requires both partners. Counseling is suggested to resolve the issue.

Q. Do my odds ever change or are they the same every month?

A. The odds are age-dependent, but nothing dramatic occurs over just a month. So postponing a procedure for a month or two will not change the prognosis in any material way.

Q. Why are multiple births so common with IVF?

A. It's because we put in more than one embryo. In some countries, there is a trend to put in just one embryo in young women as a way of avoiding multiple births.

Q. Are the chances for multiple births less with an insemination than with IVF?

A. The chances for multiples are due to the drugs used, not the insemination process. If injectable drugs are used, multiple births are possible – sometimes at an even higher incidence than with IVF.

Q. Are IVF multiple births decreasing over time as techniques improve?

A. As success rates go up, infertility specialists are putting in fewer embryos, and the multiples rate decreases.

Q. If we fail with IVF, have we reached the end of the line in terms of having a baby?

A. After an unsuccessful IVF cycle, you need to regroup and re-evaluate. Why did the cycle fail? Was there an unanticipated problem? Is there something we can change to improve the next cycle or are we doing the same thing again? Remember, regardless of how good the program is, there is no such thing as a 100 percent pregnancy rate. Perhaps a change in protocol is called for. Maybe an additional laboratory procedure is needed. This requires an extensive discussion with your IVF team and a frank assessment of the potential for future success.

Patient talk

This patient anecdote is an excellent example of the twists and turns that infertility treatments can take. This is the story of Becky and Fred. The infertility issues were hers, not his.

"I've always had some sort of female problems," Becky says. "I kept going to doctors and I wasn't getting any solutions. I pushed for more diagnostic work, but they just kept fiddling around. Things weren't getting any better. We knew we wanted children, but by this time I was about 36 years old. I was coming up to that time-clock situation. That's when I found my way to the Cleveland Clinic.

"They did X-rays and discovered a polyp in my uterus. It was removed surgically. There were also issues with some uterine fibroids and a small amount of endometriosis.

"I then started with hormone injections, and we tried to get pregnant naturally. That didn't work. Then we went to several tries with IVF and that didn't work. Along the way, I had some problems with the medication. Also, we couldn't get enough follicles to form. Finally, we got one viable egg. We went ahead, but no luck again.

"The doctors advised that with my age and what we had done so far, my odds of getting pregnant were pretty low. We decided we had had enough. We figured we're not going to have children the conventional way. I went on to have a hysterectomy and my daily life became much better."

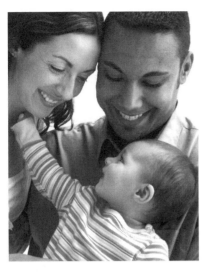

Becky and Fred had already decided that if they couldn't have children, they would adopt. Very soon after the hysterectomy surgery, they found themselves in Russia looking for children. After two trips, they came home with a little boy and a little girl.

Summary

In vitro fertilization is certainly the right answer for many people. For others, like Becky and Fred, it may not work. But they had an alternative plan already in place for that contingency. That is always a good idea.

Most, but not all, will try other approaches first. Usually these will be faster and cheaper than IVF. But often they will not provide the same success potential.

Women who are older from a childbearing standpoint might proceed directly to IVF. So, too, might a woman who is unable to tolerate the drug therapy involved in some of the lower-level treatment options.

There are important questions about your emotional and financial strength that need to be discussed and resolved with your partner before you enter an IVF program.

As you can see from the preceding pages, assisted reproductive technology has multiple variations and a great many long words and terms associated with it. What's important to remember is that you ask enough questions and gain enough understanding of the concepts to be satisfied that you are making informed choices.

The technology and techniques associated with IVF are improving all the time.

Chapter 8
Beyond In Vitro Fertilization

"Bloom where you are planted."

– *Anonymous*

There are indeed some medical steps beyond traditional in vitro fertilization. In general, these involve advanced IVF concepts.

There are women who are never able to produce good eggs. For these women, donor eggs are a possible choice. The IVF procedure would be exactly the same, but the source of the eggs would be a donor, not you. There are complex issues associated with donor programs that are addressed in Chapter 9.

Just as with women who cannot produce eggs, there are men who are never able to produce strong, healthy sperm. That being the case, a spouse's eggs might be combined via IVF with the sperm of a donor.

Then there are infertility cases that might or might not involve donors, where the woman is able to achieve pregnancy but is simply unable to sustain a healthy pregnancy. In those instances, there is an additional option – surrogacy – where somebody agrees to carry the baby for you. This is likewise a complex issue that is also discussed further in Chapter 9.

There are two additional options, which are not medically based and therefore not explored at length in this book. One is adoption. The second is to move on with your life without children, knowing that you have done all you could to have them.

Medically speaking

When no pregnancy results from an IVF cycle, there should be a mechanism to review your entire clinical case. Often a case is presented to the entire IVF team for discussion.

Following that step, a conversation should take place between the couple and a member of their IVF team to review the findings and opinions. To provide real value, this must include what can be done to improve the outcome, such as modifying the stimulation protocol, performing added laboratory techniques, or improving the uterine environment for implantation. In addition, an objective opinion as to the potential success of a subsequent cycle should be offered.

During this time when a reassessment of the IVF procedure is taking place, it is important that the couple have the support mechanism to cope with a grieving period, which all couples experience. It may be time to consult a formal therapist.

Several techniques are available that may improve the outcome in case of repetitive IVF failure. Most already have been discussed, such as assisted hatching and co-culture.

However, one exciting technique is evolving rapidly as an important option. Called preimplantation genetic diagnosis (PGD), it is worth discussing here in detail.

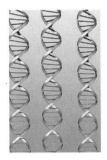

Preimplantation genetic diagnosis

As Dr. Philipson pointed out in an earlier section of this book, the potential to give birth to a baby with chromosomal problems such as Down syndrome increases with age.

When a woman reaches 42 years of age, for example, the chances of her having a baby with any chromosomal abnormality is 1 in 39. We think that is high risk. And that statistic refers only to babies who reach viability.

If we include embryos that are not viable, such as those lost in miscarriages or lost before missing a period, the frequency is even higher.

A large number of early embryos are lost without any perception that it has occurred. Fertilization of an egg with sperm occurs at midcycle and forms a "zygote." The zygote (which is the one-cell stage) starts to divide as it goes down the uterine tube. These are sometimes referred to as pre-embryos. Some of these pre-embryos will implant. These events – fertilization, formation of pre-embryos, and implantation – all occur before missing a period. Most of these embryos do not develop because of chromosomal abnormalities.

In fertility terms, this means that age-related fertility decrease is due to a chromosomal problem. Even if the embryos look perfect when examined under a microscope, many will have a chromosomal problem. It has therefore been proposed that PGD may identify these abnormal embryos so that they are not transferred. This has the potential to improve the pregnancy rate.

PGD is a process whereby a single cell is removed from the embryo and its chromosomal makeup investigated. Less commonly, two cells are removed.

The technique involves removing one cell from a day-three embryo. A hole is placed in the membrane around the embryo by exposing it to a localized area of acid or to a laser. There are typically between eight and ten cells at this stage. Removal of one cell is not thought to damage an embryo. Manipulating the embryo under the microscope is called micromanipulation, which is also not thought to harm the embryo. The chance of accidental damage to the embryo is thought to be less than 1 percent.

One other potential problem with PGD is misdiagnosis. In other words, there is always a possibility that an embryo can be diagnosed abnormal and discarded when in reality it is normal. There also is the possibility that the embryo is abnormal but diagnosed as normal and transferred into the woman.

This risk can be diminished by having further genetic testing during the pregnancy through amniocentesis (taking some of the fluid that is found around the baby) or removing a tiny piece of placenta (called a chorionic villous sampling).

It is important to understand the basic concepts of genetics.

- Each cell except the germ cells (the ovulated egg and the sperm) has 46 chromosomes. These are actually 23 pairs, one from each parent. The germ cells have 23 chromosomes. Each chromosome has two components referred to as a short (p) arm and a long (q) arm. The point between the two parts is called the centromere.

- Genes are small components of the chromosome that determine some function. Each gene is made up of series of smaller components called bases. There are four bases, frequently referenced as letters A, C, T, and G. These gene locations are often given a number. So if we say there is a mutation located at "19q13," we mean chromosome 19 at gene 13 on the long arm. This happens to be the gene for the very serious disease known as myotonic dystrophy.

- The other concept to understand is dominant trait versus a recessive trait. A dominant trait requires only one gene of the pair to be altered to show a disease. A recessive trait requires both genes of the pair to show a disease.

An embryo is analyzed for its chromosomal component. If the cell has two copies of each chromosome, it is normal.

PGD is done with specific probes that pick up numerical chromosome problems – that is, if there are more or less than two copies of the chromosomes. An abnormal number of chromosomes is called aneuploidy. We typically look for the X and Y chromosome as well as chromosomes 13, 15, 16, 17, 18, 21, and 22.

The concept of improving IVF outcome with the use of PGD is based on the belief that this procedure will pick up the embryos with abnormal number of chromosomes and these will then not be transferred.

The technique used to identify these abnormalities is called fluorescent in situ hybridization (FISH). The risk of abnormal chromosomes in delivered babies is approximately 1/400 at age 30, 1/200 at age 35, 1/60 at age 40 and 1/20 at age 45. The risk of these problems in developing embryos is far more common because most abnormal embryos result in miscarriage.

Another technique called polymerase chain reaction is used to detect single gene mutations. This technique creates multiple copies of a piece of DNA that contains the gene in question. It should be understood that many women who have PGD may not get an embryo transfer because all the embryos are abnormal with chromosomal problems.

Recurrent miscarriages

The technique of PGD is sometimes used in older women to decrease pregnancy losses.

Patients with recurrent miscarriages should be assessed for other causes before proceeding with PGD. This includes an evaluation of the uterus for congenital anomalies and an evaluation for blood-clotting disorders.

These antibody tests or blood tests for clotting disorders are not thought useful for patients who have not achieved pregnancy with IVF. They are, however, valuable for patients who have recurrent miscarriages. Genetic testing in both partners is part of the diagnosis.

If either partner carries a genetic problem, PGD can be useful. An example is that of a genetic problem called a balanced translocation. This means that the amount of DNA in the cell is normal, but its distribution is abnormal. The male and female are fine.

This usually occurs in one of the two gene copies. Each parent contributes half the DNA to the embryo. If the parent with abnormal DNA gives the good copy, the fetus is fine. If the embryo receives an abnormal copy, there could be a problem. PGD can test the embryo for this. In cases of a genetic problem in the couple, a genetic counselor definitely should be consulted.

PGD will not eliminate miscarriages from genetic problems because not all genetic problems are tested. PGD seems to be far more beneficial for women over 35 years of age with recurrent miscarriages.

Donor egg program

Patients who failed to conceive with all the infertility treatments may want to consider egg donation.

Women with an initial evaluation of poor outcome with infertility treatment may also want to consider egg donation. Research has shown that aging is more of an egg problem than a uterus problem. Therefore, as long as there is a normal uterus, pregnancy is always possible.

In a donor egg program, both the donor and recipient are evaluated. The recipient must undergo a complete medical examination that includes history of previous medical, genetic, or reproductive problems, and both a physical and psychological examination. Blood tests are performed on the recipient and partner for blood type and Rh factor, for hepatitis B and C, HIV-1 and CMV (cytomegalovirus). The women also should have rubella and varicella titer blood tests to determine whether they are immune.

Furthermore, women with medical problems may require a consultation with a high-risk obstetrics specialist who can offer an opinion about their pregnancy risk.

An egg donor can be anonymous or known. Donors are typically between the ages of 21 and 34. Some known donors are older, and the recipient couple should be aware of the increased risk of chromosomal problems and decreased fertility in using such donors. Previous history of successful fertility is ideal but not mandatory.

Donors are screened in the same way as recipients. Women at high risk for sexually transmitted disease or HIV, or women who have risk factors for certain transmissible diseases, should not be accepted into a donor program. Unlike frozen sperm, eggs are used fresh. There has never been a case of infection reported from the use of fresh eggs.

Another option for egg donation is what is called "egg sharing." As the term implies, a woman who is undergoing IVF for her own infertility problems is willing to share her eggs with a recipient in exchange for sharing the expense. Clearly, this also implies that the eggs may have an infertility problem and that, of course, only half the retrieved eggs are available to the recipient. The principal advantage is that the costs are lower.

The donor undergoes IVF as described in previous chapters. The recipient cycle is synchronized with the donor's cycle. This means starting a drug therapy at the same time as the donor and then starting the luteal phase support the day of the egg retrieval or the next day. The stimulation of the donor is done with less intensity. Usually, fewer drugs are used or another protocol is used where the total number of injections is fewer.

Cryopreserved embryo donation

Couples who have completed their family and have extra embryos frozen may choose to donate them. These are fertilized eggs and therefore are a genetically distinct form of both parents.

The selling of embryos is ethically unacceptable. Any expense should be limited to a professional fee required to facilitate the process. The embryos are quarantined for at least six months before they can be replaced. The embryo donors are then screened after the quarantine period, just as an egg donor would be screened and rejected for similar high-risk occurrences.

Donors relinquish all rights to their embryos and the recipients accept full responsibility for the children. The recipients agree to undergo the same tests as the donor.

Gestational surrogacy

Gestational surrogacy refers to the transfer of the embryo after IVF into a woman who is not genetically related to the sperm and egg donors. This procedure is infrequently used and is highly regulated in most countries in the world. Commercial (paid) surrogacy is allowed in the United States.

The indication for surrogacy is typically some medical problem such as an absent uterus or a medical condition that could result in death if pregnancy occurred. The difficulties with gestational surrogacy are legal, ethical, and religious rather than medical. The medical intervention is the same as that described for IVF and egg donation.

Front-line perspectives

Nurse-practitioner Leslie Greenhalgh, nurse-midwife Char Frires, and nurse-practitioner Suzy Pare help to run our sperm donor program.

Leslie Greenhalgh: "Sperm donors are easier to find than egg donors. Probably more than 90 percent are college students. Some get involved for altruistic reasons, but it's also easy money even though they do have to have lab tests to qualify and are tested again frequently.

"With recipient couples of donor sperm, men may feel vulnerable. They might feel less than a man. They are real quiet at first. The husband and wife have to meet with us. They also meet a counselor to discuss issues of sperm donation to ensure comfort with their decision. They do this together so they will be in agreement. Women sometimes wonder how their husband will feel about a child when it isn't his sperm. Will he feel less like a father?"

Those are big issues that deserve serious consideration by both parties.

Char Frires: "Sperm donors fill out a ten-page questionnaire and go through blood tests. Then their sperm is frozen and stored for six months because that is how long it takes to come up HIV-positive. Six months later, the lab requires them to come back again and do all the tests another time. Once they are negative twice, the lab releases the frozen sperm for use.

"My job is to support you emotionally. We know what you want and we want that, too. Our job is to help you find the way that's going to get you there and cost the least amount of money, time, and emotional, psychological, and spiritual energy."

One of the tests for women is called the Clomid Challenge Test. If that comes up abnormal, even in vitro can't help you. At that point, technology cannot give you eggs you don't have. So that tells us you need an egg donor.

Good infertility programs are very careful. They don't make it easy for a donor to get through the process. There are many reasons why egg donors are not accepted – certain types of STDs in the past, a history of difficulty getting pregnant themselves, cancer that has required radiation or chemotherapy, schizophrenia, or other serious mental illness. For every fifty applicants, programs such as ours probably approve one.

Our staff impresses on them that, yes, there is some money, but egg donors will be in a process for three to six months. They have to come in and must be available when needed. They must schedule appointments and follow through. They will go through everything that a female IVF patient does. Only the ones who truly want to do this will make it through.

Donor egg programs are even more of an emotional roller coaster than regular IVF. This is because the recipient has to depend on the kindness of strangers. But donor egg programs have even better results than IVF.

Frequently asked questions

Q. In general, who would be candidates for these advanced IVF procedures?

A. Typically, candidates would be those who have exhausted the more traditional procedures or who clearly would not be appropriate for these procedures.

Q. Are the success rates in the sperm or donor egg programs higher or lower than a traditional approach?

A. Donor egg and sperm programs have a higher pregnancy rate for a couple than traditional treatments. This is because we do this with donors who are ideal – young people with no problems.

Q. How sure are you that all the background information that donors provide is accurate?

A. We choose sources that have a track record of providing good, healthy donors who have undergone rigorous psychological screening and counseling prior to their selection.

Q. Why does an egg donor have to go through everything that a normal IVF patient experiences?

A. That's because the only way to get an egg from a woman is through IVF.

Q. How can I be supportive of my wife in all this?

A. Both of you need to be good listeners, good communicators, and just as supportive as you can be. There is no magic to this. You just need to work on it every day.

Patient talk

Joan and Rob were married in 1995. By 1997, she was taking steps to check into infertility problems. He would be the first to say he was not completely on board for a long time. Their experience is very instructive.

"We both checked out fine," Joan says. "Neither one of us had any real issues. We started with our regular doctor and just did Clomid drug therapy. Then we did an insemination. I took some drugs to stimulate more eggs. We spent about a year and a half to that point with no results.

"The years from 1997 to 2000 were devastating, sad, and lonely. I was so filled with raw emotion that I couldn't even have gone to a support group. I would have cried and been unable to talk. It is true that whenever anyone goes through anything – whether it's infertility or something else – and that no matter if you have ten people around you there is still a loneliness and an emptiness in your sadness. It was horrible.

"In 1999, I said I wanted to try in vitro. Rob didn't. That was a big bone of contention. He said all I wanted to do was spend money. We had already spent a lot and had done both inseminations and an IVF try with another hospital.

"In 1999, we found our home and we got into remodeling it. We didn't talk about our infertility for maybe a year. At the end of 2000, I told Rob that if we weren't pregnant by mid-2001, I was making an appointment with somebody. This time he said okay."

Their first consultation with the Cleveland Clinic occurred in the spring of 2001. Says Rob, "We started with one of their nurses. She was more than a nurse. She became a partner. Her confidence was infectious. She could feel our disdain for our previous experience. We were ticked. We had our walls up by the time we got to her. One day she said to us, 'Even negative people can get pregnant.'

"This nurse was the one who ultimately got our chart and called us one night to observe that whenever we had an egg and a sperm in a dish, they would never spontaneously unite. To this day, that is the only telltale sign we have as to the nature of our infertility. Somehow, my sperm does not get into her egg. That is when we went to IVF-ICSI. And that gave us our first son."

Joan picks up on the story at this point. "Rob was pulling for triplets the first time. I would have been fine with that. He said he just wanted a family. I would have been fine with five or six. We were just so desperate. However, as he now says, you learn about what makes a good pregnancy and a healthy fetus and you find out that one is the healthiest way to go."

Rob says, "For a long time, I was oblivious to what was going on. I guess I was cocky enough that I thought it was assured I could get somebody pregnant. We stood on our heads. We did it all. I was convinced it would work. I just felt it would happen in its own time. As the clock started ticking, Joan was more insistent about it. I was put off by it. I guess I was a little insulted. Part of it was bravado, but religion actually played an even bigger part."

"Everyone just wanted this so badly for us," Joan says. "People were so supportive, but after a couple of years they just didn't know what to say to us. My biggest joy now is having friends go through this and get pregnant and to be a cheerleader for them. Other people were very much cheerleaders for us." Rob adds, "Everyone being so positive in the face of my negativity was very helpful."

Joan and Rob have now gone on to have a second son via IVF-ICSI. This child unfortunately has serious health issues, including Down syndrome and extensive hearing loss. He nearly died in infancy.

Joan says, "The second child we wanted so much is a special-needs child. I believe this is our fate, that this is the design of our family. As imperfect as it may be, it is perfect. I feel this is the way it was supposed to be.

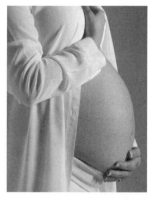

"During our pregnancy, we did share with some family and friends that genetic testing had shown this son would have Down syndrome. All of them and our doctors were always supportive. The doctor said, 'I will take care of you and this baby the best I can.' He said we had a choice to make and that he would respect that choice and be supportive whatever we did.

"Ultimately having Rob on board with me was such a relief. We were finally going through this together and not getting hung up on the cost. Once you have children, there is just nothing more awesome or perfect."

Summary

Something we say to patients is this: You never want to have to look back and know you didn't do all you felt was appropriate to reach your goal – a baby.

There may be other options for you. There may still be choices you can make. If that is so, those options and choices are at least worth a serious look before you quit.

Chapter 9
Touchy Issues

*"What one man does, another fails to do;
what's fit for me may not be fit for you."*

– Anonymous

There are many "touchy issues" associated with addressing infertility. Some religious faiths, for example, are more comfortable with infertility treatments or make more accommodations for them than others do.

Here is an example from Dr. Thomas.

"Often fertility issues relate to the timing of sexual intercourse. A married Orthodox Jewish couple is not able to start intercourse again after the wife's period until she experiences a ceremonial religious bath. Because some women ovulate early – perhaps even at the time of the bath – they are not having intercourse during ovulation. If couples are open to it, doctors can prescribe medication to shift the days of ovulation."

It is simply not possible to go through infertility treatment without confronting either religious or ethical issues. The purpose of this chapter is to help sensitize you to some of those issues and to impress upon you the need to think carefully about them. It is important to set proper expectations now.

What concerns one person may be of no concern to somebody else. That does not make one person right and another person wrong. It makes them different. One of the responsibilities of any infertility practice is to respect those differences.

If you were to put a cross section of infertility patients under a big tent, you would find great diversity:

- Different religions
- Different nationalities
- Different cultures
- Different colors

- Different family structures

- Different sexuality

- Different economic circumstances

- Different political preferences

And that pretty well describes the cross section of people who work in most large infertility practices.

When you put various dynamics together, you end up with different value systems. Under the big tent for infertility patients, there needs to be room for everyone.

We believe wherever you end up on what might be called the values continuum is okay as long as you think about the touchy issues and make decisions that will work for you both now and later. What is not okay is to ignore these issues out of ignorance or fear.

Along the way, we will provide information. We will answer your questions. But you will make the final decisions.

With respect to those decisions, we will not judge you. We will always support you.

That is such a critically important point that it bears repeating: **We will not judge you. We will always support you.**

With that said, it is now time to discuss several of the touchiest issues. You may reject some alternatives out of hand. You may elect to take considerable time to think about others. What matters is that you look at these issues before you start an infertility program and again at appropriate points after that process has started. Keep thinking about them. Keep talking about them.

Cornerstone questions

There are four fundamental questions to explore. The answers will form the foundation of what you will decide about all of the other issues associated with infertility.

Question 1: Are the two of you in agreement?

Most people we see are in a marriage or another form of committed relationship. There are certainly exceptions to that with respect to single women who join programs such as ours. But the overwhelming number of patients are part of some sort of "team."

Going through infertility treatments is one of the most stressful choices a couple will ever make. At best, it is very challenging. It has the potential to pull you together. It also has the potential to drive you apart.

Do all you can up front to ensure the two of you are on the same page. And especially if you happen to be a single woman, do all you can up front to put a solid support network in place before you go forward.

Question 2: Are your expectations realistic?

Getting pregnant, staying pregnant, delivering a healthy baby, and raising a child all take work. Where these issues are concerned, there is no "free lunch."

It has been said by many people that there are no guarantees with respect to infertility treatments. Actually, there is one thing we can guarantee. We guarantee you will experience some sort of pain along the way.

It may be physical pain from shots to stimulate egg production or from surgery to correct a blockage.

It may be emotional pain from failing yet again this month as your high hopes come crashing down.

It may be mental pain as you anguish over tough choices that result from genetic testing.

It may be financial pain as the costs continue to rise.

If your expectations are set properly today, your responses tomorrow will ease whatever pain comes your way.

Question 3: Are you okay with ART?

As you already know, ART stands for assisted reproductive technology.

The first and last words are key. In your case, you cannot achieve reproduction the traditional way. You require assistance. You require that assistance be provided in the form of some sort of technology.

There is a good chance that to achieve your goal – a baby – you will conceive in a clinical laboratory versus your own bed. Highly skilled professionals with years of training and front-line experience – supported by powerful pharmaceutical drugs and expensive equipment – are going to cause an egg and a sperm to unite in a ceramic dish.

Think about that. Do not start down this road unless you are comfortable with that concept.

Question 4: Are you patient, tenacious, and resilient?

The bad news is that there is hardly ever an infertility case where everything goes just the way you would want it to go right from the start.

The good news is that we are able to identify and address many issues. And the batting average in doing so is improving all the time.

You will quickly discover that addressing infertility often takes time – in fact, many months and sometimes years. The wrong objective is to seek a fast approach to your issues. The right objective is to work toward a good result. That is the way any responsible infertility practice will approach your situation.

With infertility, patience is more than a virtue. It is an absolute necessity.

Before you ever get to us, you have been involved in some sort of process. Perhaps you have been trying to become pregnant for a year or more and have been unsuccessful. Perhaps you are a single woman who has been wrestling with the issue of whether to become a mother. Perhaps you have been sick or become injured and have now recovered to the point where you can point your life forward again.

Whatever your situation, you have been engaged in a process. That has required some degree of patience. Now, entering an infertility program, you will have to summon your patience once again.

Of one thing you can be certain because you have already learned it – every day is not a great day when you are dealing with infertility. So you have to be not only patient, but tenacious and resilient as well. Each new day brings with it the opportunity to focus again on your goal and to continue to do whatever it takes to pursue it.

In addition to what follows, we again point you to the ASRM website (www.asrm.org), which contains many thoughtful papers on ethical dilemmas associated with infertility and its treatment.

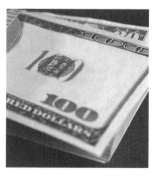

Money matters

Is making a baby your highest priority, or would you rather buy a car or redecorate your house? They all cost money. Nearly everyone has financial limits. This is an issue of priority. Understand your priorities. Talk about your priorities. Get on the same page with your priorities.

If you have an option, should you go for a lower-cost alternative that has a lower success rate or should you go with a higher-cost alternative that has a better success rate? There are levels of infertility treatment – drug therapy, insemination, in vitro fertilization. Ask the tough questions of your doctor and of each other. You are responsible for doing that. If you have options, understand them. Know the odds for people your age with your issues. Make wise choices.

Is there a point where you should quit an infertility program and move on? This is one of the toughest questions of all. It goes right back to question number four, which deals with patience, tenacity, and resilience in the face of possible continuing failure to get a good result.

Only you can answer whether you should quit. But your doctor has a responsibility to communicate clearly your chances of success and to discourage you from going beyond reasonable steps.

You owe it to yourself to base your final answer not only on your own emotions and your own opinions but also on objective information you have insisted on from your medical professionals. To the extent you can, make a fact-based decision, not an emotional decision. We recognize that is not easy.

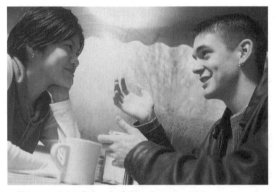

Whom to tell

Should you share your situation with your extended family such as parents or a sibling? And if you share it with some family, should you share it with all? And what about sharing it with close friends or even just anybody you happen to be talking with if the baby subject comes up naturally?

As with all the other decisions, only you can choose how transparent or how secretive you want to be.

Do you want to establish boundaries about what you are willing to discuss along the way? For example, you might tell your brother or sister that you want to start a family and have determined the only way you can do that is to get into an infertility program. As part of that first discussion, you could say something like, "I'll keep you posted with any news along the way. If I don't say anything, there's nothing to report so please don't bug me about this. I'll keep you in the loop."

Probably a good rule of thumb for most people is to be transparent with people who will be understanding and supportive and to be less so with those who do not fit that description. You want to keep yourself positive. Part of that is to get positive input from others. Spend as little time as you can around negative people and their negative attitudes.

Talking with your child

Someday, your child will ask where he or she comes from. If the child is 4 years old, the answer may be that "the stork brought you." But if the child is 14 and drills down a level or two from "the stork," there will be other choices about what you say. You need to think about that now and consider getting some counseling or advice from others who have faced this issue when it comes time for you to face it.

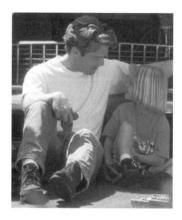

What will you say about ART? Think about that answer now. The time to provide that answer will come quicker than you think. You will get questions not only from your child, but from family and friends. You may wait fourteen years to address a question from a child, but be ready for some form of that question soon from other people.

Testing and procedure choices

There are tests or other steps in the process of addressing infertility that may run into religious or ethical considerations. Be sure to address such concerns as soon as you can. There may be options available to you.

For example, Dr. Thomas points out that some religious groups do not permit masturbation. This is the usual way that samples are collected for semen analysis or for implantation. If you belong to a religious faith that prohibits this practice, discuss optional approaches with your doctor. There may be one that will work for you.

Genetic testing

A potentially touchy issue with respect to testing relates to genetics. For the most part, children produced through assisted reproductive technology are neither more nor less susceptible to birth defects or disease than other children.

Genetic testing relates to early determination of abnormalities that produce conditions such as Down syndrome or cystic fibrosis.

HIV is another challenging issue. Increasingly, therapies are being developed to control HIV in better ways. Today, HIV is no longer an automatic dead end with respect to infertility treatment. If the HIV can be treated so that it is no longer measurable, an HIV patient has a chance to be a parent. This involves, among other things, carefully monitoring the partner as well. To lower the risk of transmission to a baby, birth is by C-section and no breast-feeding is permitted.

Nothing is automatic, but at least the door is no longer closed. An HIV patient and that person's partner need to think carefully about their situation before getting into an infertility program. But HIV in and of itself no longer prevents them from doing so.

Increasingly, new and more definitive tests will be used. Sophisticated hospitals will be dealing in advance with certain disease-inducing conditions.

With respect to genetic testing, do you in fact want to learn about potential problems such as Down syndrome in advance of your child's birth? And what would you choose to do if you received a bad testing result?

Ask two pregnant couples these questions and there is a good chance you will get two different answers.

Sex selection

During the era of the Roman Republic and subsequent imperial times, men outnumbered women. This was due in part to the practice of "exposure" of female babies to the elements. This practice of female infanticide was common. This early form of sex selection makes this topic extremely sensitive.

The role of sex selection purely for gender preference presents a significant ethical dilemma. The available procedures have obviously focused on sperm, which is the primary determinant of gender.

There are no foolproof ways to select an X or a Y sperm so as to obtain a girl or a boy. Therefore, a couple must accept the clear possibility that they will not get a guarantee of the desired gender.

Most techniques for sperm selection and insemination are proprietary and therefore no published data are available. You will have to ask your infertility center what its statistics are.

Remember, if you did nothing, you have a 50 percent chance of getting either a boy or a girl. In cases where there is a genetic disease that occurs only in a gender – typically boys – pre-implantation diagnosis will select the desired sex with almost 100 percent certainty.

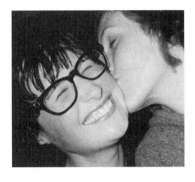

Nontraditional parenting

Single women often want to have children. We have also worked at different times with two women in a committed same-sex relationship who share that goal. In both scenarios, there is a strong desire by women to experience pregnancy, the thrill of giving birth, and the joys of parenting.

There is no question, however, that a single woman or two women in a committed relationship who choose to be parents bring with that choice certain potential complications that need to be looked at sooner rather than later. Neither approach is the traditional route to parenting. This will be a challenging choice for both you and ultimately for your children as well.

Do you have a good support network of family and friends who will stand by you during pregnancy and after you become a parent?

When your child is old enough to ask about his or her father, how are you going to respond?

Focusing on these two questions in advance is a great reality check to ensure you are doing things for the right reasons. In these two circumstances – single moms or dual moms in a committed relationship – it cannot be just about you.

Get whatever help you need to work through the tough issues that will be so important for your children.

Sperm donor issues

Let's look at the issue of sperm donation. If you use a sperm donor, you will need to think carefully about how close a match you want to your own characteristics. For some, the goal is "a baby that looks like me." For others, the goal is simply a normal, healthy baby. The closeness of the match ultimately comes down to whether the recipient plans to tell people she is a recipient.

As one of our nurse-practitioners said, "If somebody can't produce sperm and they come to us, we tell them we have to match the donor to them unless they intend to tell their family and tell this child that they used donor sperm. I give them the sperm donor list and tell them they are going to discover what their agenda is."

Sperm donation is generally anonymous, but routinely includes review of donor profiles (without names). Those profiles are descriptive with respect to donor background and characteristics. Is the donor outgoing? Does he have a strong sense of humor or is he more serious? Does he share your trait of laughing a lot?

What is your agenda? Please think about that. Like everything else in infertility treatments, make sure you are in agreement if you are a couple planning to use a sperm donor.

Egg donation

Egg donation brings with it some different twists.

Whereas sperm donation is almost always done without knowing the true identity of the donor, that is frequently not the case with egg donation. Often, there is a choice you can make to either receive eggs anonymously or from a donor you know personally.

If you use a donor you know – sibling, other family member, friend – this immediately puts into the equation a potentially complicating issue. That issue is: What relationship, if any, does the egg donor expect to have with your child? Will she be like a second mom? Does she expect to participate in decisions along the way? Will she want to be able to visit or take your child on a holiday? Or does the egg donor see her role as limited to egg donation and her expectation is that she will have no active, ongoing role in your child's life or your family's life?

That discussion and that expectation need to be addressed before you ever get into an egg donor relationship with anyone – family member or friend in particular. Everybody needs to be clear and direct and, in this instance, getting on the same page includes your spouse or partner and the egg donor if she is known to you.

And once again, as with so many other issues, now's the time to think through what you will say to your child someday.

Surrogacy

There are some women who may be able to get pregnant but cannot sustain a pregnancy. An option open to them is surrogacy. Somebody else will carry the baby and give birth.

If you determine that surrogacy is your best option, make sure you understand and accept the fact that you will have a child, but that you will do so without ever experiencing being pregnant or giving birth. Assuming that the surrogate uses your eggs and/or your spouse's sperm, there still will be a biological link.

Those are the realities. Part of electing surrogacy is that you become comfortable with all that. Surrogacy represents a large and potentially complex concept. Think long and hard about it. Make sure it works for you.

As with sperm or egg donation, discuss now how you plan to handle the inevitable questions of family, friends, and in the future, your child.

Family size

Many people come to us with a specific goal of having one child. Couples with infertility problems are often extremely pleased and grateful if they can conceive even one child.

Others come to us with a little bigger goal – perhaps two or three children if everything works out. Still others come with no goal in terms of numbers, but with the attitude that they will happily accept whatever number of children they may be able to have.

It is good to think about that issue. Where do you stand?

But it is also good to think about the broader issues that often come with fertility treatments. The reason there are so many multiple births associated with infertility treatments is that multiple eggs are often stimulated by the drug therapy we must prescribe.

How do you feel about having multiples? Understand there are higher risks to mothers and children from multiples. What is your risk tolerance? You should discuss this with your infertility specialist early in your program.

With in vitro fertilization, for example, the answer to that question will have significant bearing on how many embryos are implanted. It is far better to address that issue now to the extent it can be addressed up front than to face a possible selective reduction choice after you become pregnant.

And, with respect to extra embryos, that always raises the issue of what you want done with them. Being responsible means thinking that very sensitive issue through now – not later.

Cryopreservation

Egg freezing – a relatively new technique – will become a viable option in the future as technology improves. When that happens, egg freezing will bring additional focus to important issues such as postponing parenthood.

Freezing sperm and embryos, on the other hand, has been going on for some years already.

With respect to freezing sperm, that is often done in the case of young men who suddenly face a difficult illness such as testicular cancer or, indeed, any cancer that will require either chemotherapy or radiation treatments. Or perhaps, they have been injured in an accident. Any of these situations can have an impact on male fertility.

So some young men elect to freeze sperm for future use. All depositors in our program sign a contract, which deals with the issue of what to do with their sperm if they die. But there is also the potential issue of what to do with unused sperm if they someday use all they need and still have some left.

A companion issue relates to disposition of frozen embryos. There are today approximately half a million frozen embryos in the United States. These embryos serve as a potential source of future children for you or for somebody else.

Once you have agreed on the size of the family you want, a decision should be made about embryos that are frozen. This is often a highly emotional decision that has ethical or religious implications.

There are two options for extra embryos: donation or destruction.

The embryos can be donated to another infertile couple so that they can achieve pregnancy, or they can be donated for medical research. In addition, embryos can be transferred back into the uterus at a time when the chance of achieving a pregnancy is zero.

Many couples postpone their decision by keeping frozen embryos in storage. In addition to not facing the issue, there are annual storage fees for this.

Couples are asked by their IVF team to make this decision at the outset. Despite doing that, many couples change their mind when it is time to implement their decision.

Ultimately, the decision will be made based on your own personal belief of what an embryo is.

Many couples feel that there is a potential for life and that they will have some responsibility if their embryos are donated to another infertile couple. It is not an exaggeration to say that couples often view their embryos as sacred.

Other couples refer to these embryos as siblings of the children they may already have. Still others feel that if the embryos are donated, there may be a potential for the siblings to meet accidentally one day. And some couples believe that their embryos may have potential benefit if some disease afflicts their present children and a potential donor cannot be found.

Whatever your personal feelings may be – and we will absolutely respect those feelings – it is important to recognize that you may have to face a very difficult decision. Discuss now with your spouse or partner what you want to have done with frozen embryos if you achieve your desired family size and still have embryos in cryopreservation.

Adoption

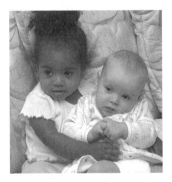

There's the possibility that you may exhaust every fertility option open to you and still not reach your goal – a baby. You now have a choice with respect to adoption.

There are many children of different ages and backgrounds in this country and overseas who can be adopted. Some are normal in the conventional sense. Some are "special needs" children.

In one sense, they all have special needs: to have parents and to be part of a family structure.

If you elect to adopt, you have many additional choices with respect to how that is done. None of these decisions should be made impulsively. That is why it is important now – before you begin infertility treatments – to begin thinking and talking about adoption as a possible alternative. It is a great choice for some people. It is not great for others. Either way is okay as long as you are in agreement with one another.

Quitting the program

Should you quit if infertility treatment doesn't seem to be working? If so, when should you do that?

Only you can make those decisions. But before you start, it would be good to look at all aspects of infertility treatment – tests, drugs, possible surgery, outcome potential, costs, and your own psychological reserve – to think about what you will do and at what point you may think about doing that.

From the standpoint of an infertility practice, your medical team has an absolute responsibility to keep you apprised of options and their prognosis. If outcome potential is very low, we have an obligation to tell you that. If it is zero, we are obligated to refuse further treatment.

Summary

As you can see, there are many touchy issues you need to confront. And for every one of those we just listed, there is probably at least one more that you might add.

Start with the four key questions.

Question 1: Are the two of you in agreement?

Question 2: Are your expectations realistic?

Question 3: Are you okay with assisted reproductive technology?

Question 4: Are you patient, tenacious, and resilient?

There is virtually no end to the touchy issues.

- Money
- Whom to tell
- Talking with your child
- Choices in tests
- Genetics issues

- Sex selection
- Nontraditional parenting
- Sperm donors
- Egg donors
- Surrogacy

- Family size
- Cryopreservation
- Adoption
- When to quit

These are all bedrock issues.

Loving a child – to say nothing of maximizing your own emotional stability – argues strongly for taking a comprehensive look at all these issues now plus whatever other items you can add to this list in the future.

You decide what's right for you. As we said earlier:
We will not judge you. We will always support you.

Chapter 10
Your Costs

> *"No guts, no glory."*
>
> – *Anonymous*

Inseminations can easily cost up to $2,000.

In vitro fertilization may well have a price tag in the $8,000 to $10,000 range.

Advanced procedures such as ICSI-IVF or the use of a donor or surrogate add even more.

Those costs will cause significant sticker shock if you are not prepared to deal with them.

On the surface, the issue of infertility costs is pretty simple.

If you have standard, middle-of-the-road health insurance, your policy will most likely address medically necessary conditions. What this usually means is that a person who needs to have a health issue fixed will find the cost is covered. Conversely, somebody who doesn't need something fixed – but merely wants something fixed solely for a purpose like infertility treatment – will find that type of procedure not covered by insurance.

There are exceptions. If, for example, you have what might be termed a high-end health insurance policy, it may indeed cover some elective procedures.

But the hard, cold fact is this: Infertility treatments are generally considered elective. Therefore, most people do not have insurance coverage for that purpose.

Case closed? Not really.

As with so many things in life, the cost issue is much more complex than you might initially think. You should really dig into this so that you maximize your potential for insurance coverage just as we encourage you to maximize your potential to get pregnant. In the process, you may well become a smarter health-care consumer and therefore better able to help yourself.

This is just one more example of the need for both of you to be in agreement. Until you actually reach that point, financial issues related to infertility will carry the potential to drive a wedge right into the family unit you are trying so hard to create and unite.

Don't give up too easily

Over time, insurance coverage can change. Companies review their health insurance programs all the time. Switching insurance vendors or changing the terms of policies happens often.

Rule 1: Get financial information up front.

This rule again addresses a key issue in infertility treatments, which is to manage your expectations.

Doing that involves much more than just having an understanding of medical treatments. It absolutely includes managing your expectations with respect to the cost of those treatments.

Who wants to deal with unpleasant conversations about money when you are in the middle of something as stressful as infertility? You don't. So get a handle on the issue of costs early in the process.

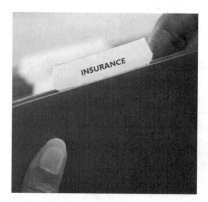

Rule 2: Understand the big picture of your health insurance.

Some provision you thought you had in your policy may disappear. Something may change. Something new may be added. If you want to owe a hospital less, you owe it to yourself to always be up-to-date about your insurance coverage.

Rule 3: Understand the little picture.

What exactly – in great detail – is covered and what is not covered by your health insurance? Yes, we know that reading insurance policies is not most people's idea of fun. Neither, for that matter, is paying unnecessarily for treatments your insurance covers and to which you are entitled if you will just take some time to look into the terms of that coverage. Ignorance is not an excuse for a bad financial decision.

A simple example of the importance of knowing the details would relate to a health insurance policy that pays zero for infertility treatments, but which pays for medically necessary diagnostic procedures. For example, you may have a blockage somewhere in your reproductive system that pertains not only to infertility, but to some other issue as well. In that case, you may well find that you are covered.

Maybe you need prescription drugs for multiple reasons – infertility being only one. You may be covered for all or at least some of them. Drug costs are a big part of the overall infertility tab. They also often represent the best opportunity to recover some of your medical costs as an infertility patient who also has other medically related conditions.

The big issue of infertility may be rejected when you knock on the door of the insurance company. But some combination of sub-issues may well be acceptable to your carrier. Keep probing. Keep pushing. Be your own best advocate. If you don't advocate for yourself, who will?

Rule 4: Get the best information you can.

Every large infertility practice will have a financial counselor. A key part of that person's job is to provide you with understandable information. A second key element of the job is to answer your questions – early. It is important for you to insist on both of those things happening.

But that person is not your only good source of information. Chances are you also have a benefits administrator where you work. That person has the same responsibilities as an infertility practice financial counselor – to provide understandable information and give clear answers to your questions. Have an in-depth conversation with your benefits administrator at the outset. Get your questions answered right away. Stay in touch along the way.

An additional resource is, of course, the insurance company itself. Going online and using the phone are effective ways to mine good information from your insurance company for the purpose of helping you to avoid nasty surprises.

Talking with a financial counselor

Dennis Lord is the financial counselor for our infertility practice. Every day, he deals with families and individuals going through infertility treatments. His perspective on the financial side of infertility merits your close attention.

"Some people think infertility treatments are just for the wealthy. That is not correct. Most of the people we see for in vitro fertilization, for example, are what would be classified as middle-income.

"Get all the facts. Ask all the questions you want. Make sure there are no hidden costs or potential surprises.

"People who come to us are very serious about going through this process. There are many sources for money for them to pay for this, and we are familiar with all of them.

"Patients use credit cards or home equity loans. Some borrow against their 401-K or profit-sharing accounts. Lots of people apply their flexible spending accounts for medical expenses and take tax deductions for this. We can't give you tax advice, but we can advise that you check with your own tax advisor to look into whether you can take medical deductions for your infertility procedures.

"There are some insurance policies that pay for the diagnostic work-up, or at least part of that. Where many insurance companies draw the line in the sand is when the diagnostic phase evolves directly into infertility treatments. Check with your insurance administrator. Read your policy. Ask questions. Know the codes we use for billing. Do your homework. Understand that where insurance coverage stops is where most infertility practices will require money up front from that point on.

"It's important for patients to look at the issue of costs as early as possible. We need to have a mutual understanding about costs and insurance coverage. We always try to address these matters very early in a relationship. Lots of times patients are not comfortable discussing these matters with their insurance companies. In those cases, we contact the company or the patient's own company benefits people on their behalf.

"Infertility patients would be well advised to ask these questions when they talk about their issues with a financial counselor.

- Will you get into these matters with my insurance company on my behalf?

- Will you contact my company benefits administrator for me?

- Do you offer some sort of payment plan?

- Do you require payments up front?

- How much do the drugs cost and do you think some portion of those might be covered?

- What about the diagnostic tests and possible coverage for those?

"It is just so important for people to understand their costs up front so they are prepared in advance."

The bottom line

Earlier, we had a chapter on "Preventing Infertility from Happening to You." Hand in glove with that is the parallel need to prevent unhappy financial surprises from happening to you.

Please do not let this issue drag on. Make sure you get to a point of being comfortable with the costs, or at least reach a point where you are less uncomfortable.

Nobody likes to talk about dollars. But you just have to bring yourself to do that. Now.

Avoid the temptation to shop price. Good infertility practices are expensive. But they also offer the best hope to reach your elusive goal – a baby.

The hope is that your infertility treatment experience will be one of those times you can look back on and know you worked with very good people who helped you have the best possible chance.

Patient talk

This story is about Cindy and her experiences.

"I was an only child and always dreamed about having a large family.

"In our case, it was a fourteen-year journey from the first treatment until finally giving birth.

"We tried lots of approaches. My husband had issues. His sperm count was okay, but he had low motility. So he had to go through some surgery for a varicocele problem [dilation of the veins around the testicles] and that really didn't help at all. I had problems with undersized babies and miscarried four times over the years – twice with inseminations, once from a spontaneous pregnancy, and once with an IVF pregnancy. It was the same every time – underweight babies where the heartbeat would stop. Nobody could pin down the cause.

"We tried everything. Ultimately, I was referred to one of the top high-risk pregnancy specialists in the country. She was able to pin down the cause – these babies were not being properly nurtured in my uterine cavity. They were not getting the blood supply they needed to grow and develop as normal, healthy babies. She got that turned around with something as basic as aspirin therapy.

"I got pregnant again for the fifth time – this time by IVF. It was a very difficult pregnancy. I was toxemic. I had pre-term labor. I ended up hospitalized and subsequently at home in bed for nearly all of my third trimester. Despite all that, I think being pregnant and giving birth was the best experience of my life.

"As to the best advice I would give somebody else, it's this: Don't look for magic answers. Find a really good infertility center. Be persistent. Follow your dream. My dream was to become pregnant and give birth. It took a long time, but I got there.

"My insurance didn't cover much of this at all. It did cover some of the infertility treatment, but I have a policy with a $10,000 lifetime cap for infertility.

"I would have done anything. We have spent a ton of our own money – more than $100,000 over the years. I didn't care how much it cost. I just wanted to be a mom."

Summary

Most people will never spend anywhere near that amount. But this case history clearly shows there can be significant out-of-pocket expense for anyone who pursues this dream.

One more time: It is essential to go into infertility treatment with your eyes wide open from a financial standpoint.

Chapter 11

The Emotional Roller Coaster of Infertility

"Hope is grief's best music."

– Anonymous

It is clear that infertility treatment is really not something over which you can exert the same control as you can in your daily life.

That is hard for many people to accept because just taking the step to enter an infertility program is an indication that a person likes to be in control.

Obviously, in doing that, you are seeking help to bring a problem under control. Far less obviously, you have only limited control of the eventual result. That's a fact. Ultimately, you are not in control of the desired outcome – an egg and a sperm uniting to create a baby.

So if you cannot control the outcome, where should you focus your energy? The answer is to learn to control how you respond to what happens and focus on stress-relieving options for quality of life.

You may not control the process, but you definitely can take steps to make sure you are supported as you go through that process.

Learn to accept your emotional responses to infertility issues and the elements of your program that address those issues.

Learn to notice your reaction to your own impatience for quick results.

Learn to grieve fully any lack of success, and love yourself as you are.

Learn to improve how you respond to a spouse who is dealing with his or her own emotional issues just as you are dealing with your issues.

Accomplishing these goals will bring you face to face with three powerful emotions that are almost certain to be part of your makeup during the process.

Anger

When it comes to infertility, life is simply not fair.

Why is it that a good person like you – a person who will be a loving parent – cannot get pregnant? That is not fair.

Why is it that other people who are irresponsible and perhaps even abusive have children and you have not been able to do so? Why is it that people who do not value children can have them and somebody like you, who values them so highly, cannot have children?

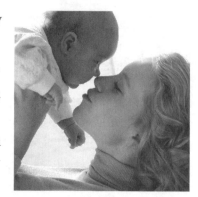

There is often a great deal of anger associated with infertility. If these feelings are present in you or your spouse, you should deal with them as part of addressing your infertility.

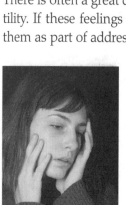

Grief

Chronic failure to get pregnant is what has brought you to us in the first place. You are already at some stage of grief before you ever arrive at the doorstep of an infertility clinic.

Every subsequent month you fail brings with it a sense of loss. Loss equals grief.

Just as with anger, if you are grieving you need support.

Hope

If anger and grief weigh heavily on infertility patients, hope is what keeps you going.

Every month is a new opportunity to succeed.

Every medical option available to you is a new, potential solution to your infertility.

Every day is yet another chance to strengthen relations with your spouse. Remember, infertility is a couple's problem.

When it comes to emotions, the job description for an infertility practice is this: We help you deal with your anger and grief so your energy can be focused on hope.

Hope is what brings you back. Hope is what keeps you in the program. Hope is what drives you forward. Hope is what helps you overcome anger and grief.

Facilitating hope

In a general sense, we expect every staff person associated with our program to be an advocate for hope.

We look to all of our people to create not only a superb professional environment but a relentlessly positive environment as well – an environment where hope can truly flourish.

Yes, we will tell you the truth. No, we will not raise your hopes unrealistically. But there is an important difference between periodic reality checks and pervasive negativity. A reality check is okay. Pervasive negativity is not.

We want you to succeed. Ultimately, we want you to leave us believing you tried every reasonable option in accordance with your values. We want you to go forward stronger for having gone through the experience – even (perhaps especially) if you cannot meet your goal.

That is what we hope. One of our most important jobs is to be facilitators for what you hope. One of the elements of remaining hopeful is to understand and deal with both the medical and emotional stresses that inevitably result from addressing infertility.

Medically speaking

Even for a couple who successfully conceives, there are higher than normal rates of anxiety during pregnancy. And postpartum depression is common. In women who experience multiple births, the rates of postpartum depression exceed those of women who experience single births.

Another important issue to consider that is particularly sensitive for women who have multiple births is the potential for a bigger workload combined with an increasing feeling of social isolation because of all you must do and the limited time you have to accomplish it. It is critical for all couples to be prepared for these types of problems and to seek help immediately if they occur.

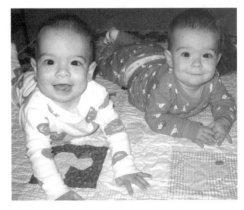

Psychologically speaking

How many times have we been told this? "If you would just relax, this would happen."

There is certainly no medical proof to support that.

But there is plenty of medical proof to support the statement that infertility and the ability to relax are often like oil and water. Cynthia Austin, M.D., an infertility specialist on our staff, has this to say: "I am not sure if stress causes infertility, but I know infertility causes stress. We believe it is important for patients to deal with the stresses they're facing. Usually their resistance fades after the first appointment."

With that in mind, please pay close attention to the advice that follows from two of our counselors.

Dana Brendza, Psy.D., is a psychologist on our hospital staff who specializes in dealing with patients and the stresses and other emotional issues caused by infertility.

Now the mother of two, she knows a great deal about these issues. Yes, she studied them. But she also miscarried four babies herself at approximately the three-month point of pregnancy. She has experienced her own anger and grief. Dr. Brendza knows the importance of hope.

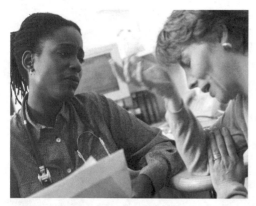

"Every day, patients come in who are in their late 30s and didn't realize they would have so much trouble. A lot of us focused on a career and married later. It ended up being kind of late for us to have children because of the way our lives unfolded.

"My own experience was really, really devastating. The older you get, the more you think you may not be able to have children. What happened to our family enables me to understand on a very personal level what others are going through. I want to help people with these problems because I have been through some of this myself.

"We see a lot of patients with depression and anxiety. When people first come to us, they feel like they're being evaluated and that we could potentially stop the in vitro process. They don't want to admit flaws. We want to reassure them right away that we're not here to stop the process. We're here to help make the process go as well as it possibly can.

"We try to determine if our patients are experiencing depression or anger they need to deal with. Is infertility stressing their marriage? Is the cost creating a financial strain? Are they upset because there are no guarantees with infertility treatments? Is their spouse likely to end the marriage if it is childless? All of these situations require support.

"It's important not to hide things. We want you to have a good outcome, to enjoy the baby you tried so hard to have, and to be able to cope with taking care of that baby. We are part of the process of helping you reach your goals.

"In my practice, I meet a lot of people who are going to be recipients of egg or sperm donation. But it is certainly not limited to that scenario. Regardless of your issue, it's not enough for us just to meet the woman. We like to meet the couple. We want to get a sense of where each one is.

"How eager is each partner to be in the program? Are they both entering into this willingly? Have they thought through any religious or ethical issues they may have? Do they plan to discuss this with their family? What about their friends? At an age-appropriate time, what do they plan to share with a child?

"A good example of an issue that requires careful discussion relates to egg donors. We require the recipient to come in to meet with us. It's one thing if the egg donor is anonymous. She will relinquish all rights, the recipient won't know much about her, and she won't have any future contact with the family. It is quite another thing if the egg donor is a family member or close friend. In those cases, we also require the donor to meet with us for evaluation.

"Does the donor consider her eggs as genetic material she is giving as if she were donating a kidney or does she view her eggs as her own children? Does she see potential offspring as her biological offspring? For us, that would be a red flag. We would probably steer that donor away from doing it. It might just be too hard for her to let go.

"The response I like to hear from a donor is that 'I am doing this as an act of goodwill. I do not consider this my child. I consider it cells that I am donating. It's a gift. I am not carrying this baby. The recipient is the mother. If my sister or friend someday decides to tell the child about me, I will keep an appropriate distance. If the family wants me to know the child, I will do that. But I will consider it my relative or friend's child, not my child.' That would be a healthy response. That process should go forward.

"Most donor egg recipients feel they are connected to the baby because the donated egg is put in them and they experience the pregnancy. They may be a little sad their own genetic material is not passed on, but at least the experience of being pregnant and giving birth partially makes up for that.

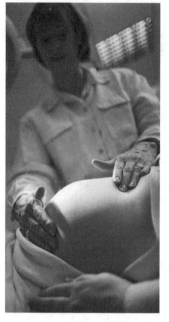

"Our goal is one healthy, full-term, good-weight baby. Twins are a handful. You really need a family and support system. I don't think we would ever encourage a goal of having more than twins. But every time you implant more than one embryo, there is always the chance for twins. And even with one, it can split into twins. So we like to assess how realistic people are about a potential multiple birth.

"Another issue is how much information to share with others. Sometimes other people aren't good about protecting your boundaries or perhaps they are very critical of choices you make.

"Depending on your own family situation, some-times it is better to keep certain things private. For example, some people who are getting donor eggs talk to family members or friends about in vitro fertilization but choose not to mention the egg donor piece. They may think it's simpler not to tell. They may believe the other person wouldn't be able to handle that information. Or perhaps they feel a grandchild might be treated differently if grandparents don't feel a genetic connection to the grandchild.

"There's an ongoing disagreement in our field about what to disclose about being a donor egg recipient. Some psychologists think it is better not to tell your family or child about any of this. Others find it is best to be honest about every-thing and to at least tell the child when it is age-appropriate to do so. Regardless of how you may feel about these difficult issues, you need strength to make good choices that work for you and your family. We are here to help you do that.

"Please don't be afraid to seek professional help for your anxiety or depression. It's common to experience those things in the midst of treatment for infertility. Let people know what you are going through. Reach out to those who are clos-est to you. You may even want to share it with somebody in your workplace. If you are a religious person, use your belief system to maximum advantage. Don't go through all of this alone."

Hanging tough

In the very first chapter, we talked about the need to blend all of the scientific and medical issues with "matters of the spirit." We used three words: Commitment. Perseverance. Confidence.

Those are more than just words. Dealing with infertility – hopefully defeating it – requires more than just science and medicine. It is true we will treat all your technical issues. But that is not enough.

Our objective is to treat the whole person.

Lynne Norrie, RN, MSN, is another member of our infertility practice. She is a clinical nurse-specialist with three well-developed specialties that she brings to our work.

1. Preventive mental health for childbearing families.

2. Mind/body therapy for improving the reproductive health of women.

3. Group psychotherapy for specific populations, including infertility patients.

Like Dr. Brendza, she is central to our goal of treating the whole person.

Ms. Norrie asks, "How do you maintain hope?"

She says, "Hope is within all of us. I have hope for everybody. I promise nothing, but I always say, 'I hope.' My job is to help our patients reach their own hope."

Ms. Norrie helps you do whatever it takes to find and sustain hope. This begins with listening to you. On the other end of the spectrum, it may ultimately include recommending something like guided imagery CDs to help you visualize success in conceiving, maintaining your pregnancy, giving birth, and raising a child.

"People find hope in many ways. We have to get to know the unique woman and her strengths. Some patients might say to us, 'I'm a failure.' It's important for them to change that thinking to believe that 'I deserve to be a parent.' That does not mean you will succeed in having a biological child, but it does mean you know you deserve to reach that goal. This type of thinking will help you maintain your hope even if the process isn't working for you at a particular point in time.

"An exercise I do with couples is called 'active listening.' I try to help couples really hear each other. One might want to tell their parents they are in an infertility program; the other might not want to do that at all. Perhaps we can help a couple find a compromise such as one speaking about infertility treatment with the family only when the other one is not present. They both deserve support. We just have to find ways to help them hear their partner. Then it is easy for them to find creative solutions.

"I see lots of individuals with ethical dilemmas. I have them talk about those dilemmas in relation to their belief system, their faith, or whatever resource they use to come to decisions they will be able to live with comfortably. So basically, wherever the couple is when they get here is where I start. We determine why they're here and what they want to learn.

"We work with patients and couples on their issues and also in small group settings where they can reach out to others going through the same process.

"I see people who choose not to talk about their grief very often, but they make a beautiful memorial garden or perhaps they express how they feel through art. I trust everyone's own process is right for them at that moment. We just try to find ways to support their process and maybe expand it in little ways. Grief is energy and it needs to flow. Families need to refuel their energy throughout this difficult process.

"Expanding your options to express yourself and knowing yourself better are not only an important part of addressing fertility but will have a carryover benefit that will help you for the rest of your life.

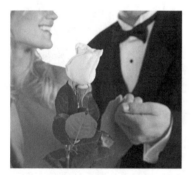

"Do your priorities match your commitments?

"What are you doing to strengthen as a couple to be more open to giving and receiving love?

"Those are two good questions to review not only for infertility purposes, but for almost anything you might be doing."

Everyone has a story

There is no cookie-cutter solution for infertility patients. Hasn't that become evident as you read about the experiences of the patients who are profiled in this book?

Every story is different. Every circumstance is different. Every person needs to be treated individually.

"I start by making an assessment of the couple," says Ms. Norrie. "I ask them about their strengths. What strengths do you have as a couple? Maybe their strength is good communication or a sense of humor. For others, it may be common interests or complementary skills. A healthy couple has flexibility in their roles, shares common interests, and can communicate their feelings to each other. In counseling patients, we tap into the abundance of strengths they have.

"Then I listen to their story. I honor every story. Everyone has significant and special factors in their history.

"I ask patients what they've done to help themselves, where they are in the process, and what they feel brought them to me.

"There's a wide range of responses. For some, they are overwhelmed with sadness. Others may be withdrawing from their partner. The couple may not be in agreement on how to cope while facing their infertility. Many come to me because they are having difficulty with family or friends they feel are pressuring them. Others have religious or ethical concerns. Families come that are wrestling with spiritual matters heightened by a medical process that is challenging their belief systems.

"There are many people having trouble dealing with their own grief and who find themselves also feeling responsible for managing the grief of other family members. These people say they are constantly being asked, 'Are you pregnant yet?' Every month they have a recurrent loss. I teach them how to say, 'Thank you for your interest and caring, but would you mind letting us get back to you when we have something to share?' That gives them a little space.

"Cost is a big issue for many people. They ask, 'When should I quit? When is enough?' I don't answer that question. I can't. But I help them tap into their own wisdom. This all involves a mind-body-spirit connection. At the end of the day what I help people do is to access the wisdom of their own hearts to get some signs about what is best for them.

"The emotions I see most often are sadness and anger. Those are both components of the grieving process. There can be recurring grief in infertility. If you have a diagnosis for cancer, you have the initial shock and grief. After that, you are often on your way to getting better. With infertility, you can have recurrent grief every month. That wears people down. It can stress relationships.

"I often say there are no negative side effects from getting calmer. I don't think that is all people need to do. But I do know getting calmer will help people with the quality of their life generally and with respect to infertility treatment specifically. The last thing we want is for somebody to get pregnant, then divorced. Don't do all the infertility work and then not have a marriage left. So I very much see the focus of my work as helping improve the quality of patients' lives wherever they are in the process."

Stress hardiness overview

Over time, Lynne Norrie has developed what she calls Ten Stress Hardiness Suggestions for Couples in Infertility Treatment. Here is her recommended process:

"Couples in our infertility program quickly come to understand that there is grief associated with the fact their bodies are not working as they had hoped.

"That grief brings with it symptoms of both physical and emotional tension, and often spiritual dilemmas.

"This stress is further compounded by economic and time crunches as well as the emotional roller coaster of menstrual cycles and medications.

"Many couples are surprised to experience a spiritual dilemma where they question their beliefs. Some also have relationship issues within both the couple and also with their family and friends.

"For most people, this accumulation of stresses is very difficult to manage. These potentially overwhelming stresses are the main reason that our infertility team recommends that families make a determined effort to raise their level of 'stress hardiness' early in a treatment program.

"To help with that, we have created a list of self-care activities that have been shown to be helpful.

"Hopefully, you will select several of these self-care options that you believe would be helpful and easy to implement in your family."

Four strategies for couples

Couple's Strategy 1: Increase the "everyday kindness" you do for each other and create a set time to listen to each other lovingly.

Couple's Strategy 2: Meet other couples with infertility issues by attending monthly Resolve meetings. (Readers, please note that information on the organization Resolve and its programs for couples with infertility is included in Chapter 12 – Helpful Resources.)

Couple's Strategy 3: If prayer is within your belief system, establish a prayer ritual to ready you for parenthood and to align yourself with spirit, spend time with inspirational reading or tapes, or play music during reflection.

Couple's Strategy 4: As a couple, look at your total life activities and choose how you can temporarily reduce those that are stressful and bring little enjoyment. Use your power to free up time and energy for this process.

Six strategies for individuals

Individual Strategy 1: If medically appropriate, increase your regular exercise routine or begin a stretching and brisk walking regimen. (Be sure to consult your doctor about this first.) Also, increase your rest and sleep, through naps or getting to bed earlier.

Individual Strategy 2: Listen to relaxing music at key transitions in your day. Also, include focused breathing of a full "in breath" and a fully released "out breath." This will bring you to what we call your anchor.

Individual Strategy 3: Purchase a journal and write from your heart several times a week.

Individual Strategy 4: Use positive self-talk to combat fearful thoughts. "I deserve to be a parent" is one thought that is calming.

Individual Strategy 5: Learn something new. Don't put your life on hold. Do something new and different that is both interesting and enjoyable.

Individual Strategy 6: Speak to your physician or nurse if you believe your symptoms are not improving and it is therefore becoming more difficult to function in your daily life. You deserve support!

These ten strategies (four for couples and six for individuals) are important to creating stress hardiness.

Use all of your tools

Life gives each of us a toolbox full of helpful ways to shape how we live and how we react to what comes our way. There are few times in your life when you will have greater need for those tools than during an infertility program. One of the choices you will make is how many of those tools to use.

If you want to experience the smoothest possible journey through the uncertainties of infertility, the best advice we can give you is to experiment with every one of those tools and commit to the ones that increase your sense of well-being.

Patient talk

This is Rachel's story.

"I had really difficult periods for a long time – lots of pain and bleeding. I was missing days of work every month.

"My gynecologist suggested I have a laparoscopy to see if we could find out was wrong. It turned out I had endometriosis. I had surgery to address that problem. I had really bad endometriosis in my uterus and also all over my intestines, which is why I was having stomach problems. I was told that my problem in getting pregnant was that my uterine wall was so scarred from the endometriosis that the sperm could not get where they needed to go. But tests also showed my fallopian tubes were open and that I was ovulating.

"It was suggested that we try some inseminations accompanied by the use of Clomid. At this point, we had tried everything but IVF. The only thing I ever wanted in my entire life was children. All of a sudden I thought I was never going to have them. I had to go on an antidepressant.

"Eventually, I had to go to IVF. The first time, I was scared to death, completely stressed out. I ended up with hyper-stimulation syndrome and also not real good eggs on this first try. I had to take pain pills and had some nasty side effects. I was completely devastated when it didn't work. I really questioned if I wanted to spend that kind of money again.

"I had decided not to try again, but my parents gave me the support to do so. The second time, the doctors adjusted the drugs, I got better eggs, and I got more eggs. It worked.

"Ultimately, I was divorced before I became a mother. Today, I'm a single parent.
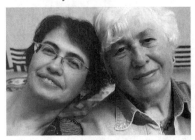
My mom went with me to every information appointment, helped me choose a sperm donor, and even went to psychological counseling with me. Some other people in my family also helped pick the donor.

"My father was the only one who initially had a problem with what I was doing. He questioned bringing a child into the world without a father. Today, he tells everyone about it. I now have two IVF children. My dad went with me for the second procedure – both for the egg retrieval as well as subsequently to watch the actual implant.

"Today, I still think about bringing a child into the world without a father. But I look at a lot of other situations, and I know my children are more loved and taken care of than a lot of children in two-parent families.

"I would love to be married, but I was not willing to do what is called 'settle.' I just never met the right person. But I am now a very happy unmarried person. I am so happy and so fulfilled at this point in my life with these children that this is all I need and all I want.

"I'm beginning to network with other professional women in my area who have also become mothers through use of donor sperm. We're doing this for our children so that when they're teenagers, they can get together with other kids and say, 'Can you believe what our mothers did?' I want my children to know there were other kids conceived like they were."

Summary

Truly, infertility treatment can be an emotional roller coaster.

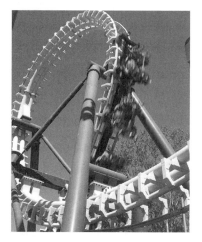

Let go of control in a traditional sense. Put that energy into strengthening yourself as you go into the infertility process. Be kind to yourself so you are able to be both patient and persistent. Use hope to manage your anger and grief.

Remember, your spouse is experiencing his or her own emotional roller coaster. It is not easy for either one of you.

Often, people see reaching out to a counselor as a sign of weakness. In fact, doing that is a sign of strength.

Keep thinking about that great quote in this chapter: "There are no negative side effects from getting calmer."

Chapter 12

Helpful Resources

> *"For knowledge is itself power."*
> – *Sir Francis Bacon*

There are multiple resources that can help you. And there are many that may be less than helpful.

We want you to know how to use our hospital and our practice as one of those helpful resources. Information on how to do that is included in this chapter.

Beyond that, we also are listing information on several other organizations. By and large, we are taking this information directly from their own materials in their own words.

We are always careful when we suggest a patient may want to access information from somebody else. The inclusion of these additional websites in this book should give you confidence that we think these organizations and their information are very credible.

At this point, we again want to send up a red flag with respect to some of what can be found on the Internet. Infertility is a health issue that inspires great emotion. Some of the information about it is good. Some is bad. Please be careful that you do all you can to know the difference.

We strongly recommend that you use other people in your life for day-to-day support and that you depend on your doctor for medical information. Your doctor is not going to suggest you stand on your head or go on some fad diet if you want to get pregnant. On the other hand, it is possible that some "helpful" person on the Internet might tell you to do just that.

American Fertility Association

Website: www.theafa.org

The AFA is a national organization dedicated to assisting women and men facing decisions related to family-building and reproductive health.

American Society for Reproductive Medicine

Website: www.asrm.org

Among ASRM's helpful services are a high-quality website and a wide range of useful publications about many areas of reproductive medicine and infertility. These publications – like this book – have been written for you, not medical professionals.

The ASRM is an organization of close to 9,000 physicians, researchers, nurses, technicians, and other professionals dedicated to advancing knowledge and expertise in reproductive biology. Affiliated societies included the Society for Assisted Reproductive Technology, the Society for Male Reproduction and Urology, the Society for Reproductive Endocrinology and Infertility, and the Society of Reproductive Surgeons.

American Urological Association

Website: www.auanet.org

The AUA is the premier professional association for the advancement of urological patient care. Useful information from AUA available on the Internet includes male infertility factors and the management of those conditions.

Centers for Disease Control and Prevention

Website: www.cdc.gov

The CDC is part of the United States Department of Health and Human Services. Its website is a resource for statistics and other information about infertility. The statistics include data on leading infertility clinic success rates.

The Cleveland Clinic

Website: www.clevelandclinic.org.

If you wish to go directly to information on in vitro fertilization, use this website address: www.clevelandclinic.org/ivf/lab.

If you wish to access the website for male factor infertility, go to www.clevelandclinic.org/ivf/male.

The Cleveland Clinic has long been ranked as one of the premier medical facilities in the United States. This recognition includes specialties related to supporting infertility patients – gynecology, urology, and psychiatry. The physicians and staff of the Cleveland Clinic live by the motto "Every Life Deserves World-Class Care."

fertileHOPE

Website: www.fertilehope.org.

This is a nonprofit organization dedicated to helping cancer patients faced with infertility. If you are a woman or a man with cancer history and you aspire to reproduce, fertileHOPE is an organization that can provide helpful information.

Resolve

Website: www.resolve.org.

Resolve is a nationwide nonprofit network of chapters mandated to promote reproductive health and to ensure equal access to family-building options for men and women experiencing infertility or other reproductive disorders. Resolve also provides support services and physician referral and education. These services include an infertility specialist physician registry and a toll-free help line.

Resolve sponsors a support group at our hospital for couples experiencing infertility. This group meets regularly. We recommend you find out whether there is a Resolve chapter in your area.

Chapter 13
Glossary of Terms

> *"The first step is the hardest."*
> – *Anonymous*

Yes, the first step is the hardest. But take that step. Do it today.

Along the way, you don't need to memorize all the fancy medical terms. But you do want to have enough of a handle on your situation that you get the concepts.

We have divided this chapter into two sections:

1. Eighteen terms you simply have to know. No excuses.

2. Other terms you may want to look up, but there is no need to commit any of those to memory.

Let's start with that first small group of absolutely essential terms:

18 essential terms

Assisted reproductive technology (ART): This term includes all procedures that try artificially to induce a pregnancy (such as insemination).

Conceive: To achieve a pregnancy.

Cryopreservation: The storage of eggs, ovarian tissue, sperm, testicular tissue, or embryos by a freezing process.

Donor: A person who voluntarily gives sperm, eggs, or embryo to another person.

DNA: The genetic material in a cell.

Egg: The gamete of a woman (also called an oocyte).

Embryo: The result of fertilization of an egg by a sperm. An embryo develops into a baby.

Fertilization: The process whereby a sperm transmits its genetic material into an egg and then subsequently develops into a cell with a different genetic material from the contributing egg or sperm.

Follicular phase: The days of the cycle from menstruation to ovulation.

Follicle: The basic unit in the ovary that contains an egg.

Hormones: Chemicals in the body that allow communication from one gland to another. For example, the pituitary gland in the brain communicates with the ovary or testicle using a hormone called FSH.

Infertility: The inability to conceive after one year of unprotected intercourse.

Insemination (IUI): Placement of ejaculated sperm in the reproductive tract of a woman by artificial means. The sperm can be placed in the cervix or uterus. The latter is referred to as intrauterine insemination (IUI).

In vitro fertilization (IVF): Fertilization of an egg by a sperm outside the body.

Luteal phase: The days of the cycle from ovulation to the day before menstruation (full flow) occurs.

Ovulation: Release of an egg from the ovary.

Sexually transmitted disease (STD): A disease that is passed by sexual contact.

Sperm: The carrier of genetic material ejaculated by the male.

Other terms

Agglutination: Clumping of cells.

Agonist: A drug that elicits the same initial reaction as a natural hormone.

Amniocentesis: The procedure that takes some fluid from around the fetus for the purpose of genetic analysis.

Ampullae: The area of the uterine tube (also called the fallopian tube) where fertilization occurs.

Andrology: The specialty that deals with male infertility.

Aneuploidy: Abnormal genetic material.

Antagonist: A drug that blocks the action of a hormone.

Antral Follicle Count (AFC): The number of follicles, the basic unit in the ovary that contains an egg.

Anovulation: No spontaneous development or release of an egg.

Autoimmune: An immunological response against one's own body.

Azoospermia: Absence of sperm in the ejaculate.

Basal Body Temperature Test: The first morning temperature, which is usually the lowest in the day.

Body Mass Index (BMI): A formula where weight is related to height. The BMI number tells us whether the weight is outside the normal range.

Chlamydia: A bacterium that causes a sexually transmitted disease.

Chromosome: The structure in the nucleus of the cell that contains the genetic material called DNA.

Clomid Challenge Test: This is used to assess ovarian reserve. This involves two blood tests. The patient is also given the drug clomiphene. The first blood test is before taking the drug, the second after completing the five-day course of clomiphene.

Controlled ovarian hyperstimulation (COH): The use of drugs to stimulate the ovary to produce an increased number of eggs.

Ectopic pregnancy: Pregnancy that occurs outside of the normal location – the uterus.

Endocrinology: The study of hormones.

Endometriosis: The presence of the glands that are normally found in the uterus outside of the uterine location.

Estradiol/estrogen: The principal hormone produced by the ovary.

Fibroids/myomas: Growths or benign tumors in the uterus.

Follicle: The structure in the ovary that contains the egg, which is microscopic.

Follicle-stimulating hormone (FSH): The hormone produced by the pituitary gland in the brain, which affects the growth of the egg and production of hormones by the ovary.

Gonorrhea: A bacterium that causes a sexually transmitted disease.

Gonadotropin: A hormone or drug that affects the production of hormones or development of an egg or sperm. The term applies to FSH/LH specifically.

GIFT: Gamete intrafallopian transfer. This is the placement of an egg and sperm into the uterine tube by a surgical procedure.

Hirsutism: Excessive facial or body hair in a woman.

Hypothalamus: The portion of the brain that controls the pituitary gland.

Hysterosalpingogram (HSG): An X-ray procedure that includes the injection of dye to evaluate the tubes and uterus.

Hysteroscopy: The insertion of a small-caliber camera into the uterus to evaluate the cavity.

Impotence: The inability to achieve an erection.

Inhibin: A hormone produced by the testicle or ovary to provide "feedback" to the pituitary gland.

Intracytoplasmic sperm injection (ICSI): A procedure where a single sperm is injected into an egg.

Laparoscopy: A procedure where a small camera is inserted into the abdomen to visualize the pelvic organs. Some surgical repairs can be accomplished by laparoscopy.

Luteinizing hormone (LH): A hormone produced by the pituitary gland that controls hormone production by the testes or ovaries.

Libido: Sex drive.

Microsurgery: Surgery performed with the use of a microscope.

Morphology: The appearance of the sperm, egg, or embryo. For sperm, the results are usually reported as a percentage. In eggs, morphology is assessed by the stage of development. Embryos are assessed by several criteria such as symmetry of cells.

Motility: The number of sperm that are moving normally.

Oligospermia: Low sperm count.

Ovarian hyperstimulation syndrome (OHSS): Excessive stimulation of the ovaries in response to ovulatory drugs.

Pelvic inflammatory disease (PID): Inflammation of pelvic organs such as tubes and ovaries. Acute PID is the result of infection and chronic PID is probably secondary to a previous infection and is usually seen as damage to the tubes and as scar-tissue formation.

Pituitary gland: The gland in the brain that controls the ovary through the production of FSH/LH.

Polycystic ovary syndrome (PCOS): A medical problem that is characterized by irregular periods and excessive hair or acne and possibly the appearance on ultrasound of very small cysts in the ovary.

Polyp: The presence of a growth (usually benign) in the cavity of the uterus.

Pre-implantation genetics (PGD): The procedure whereby a cell is removed from the developing embryo that is growing in a petri dish. This is done to assess genetic makeup.

Progesterone: A hormone produced by the ovary after ovulation or by the placenta.

Retrograde ejaculation: Ejaculation of semen in whole or in part into the bladder.

Selective reduction: Reducing the number of embryos by an ultrasound-guided procedure in a woman where multiple gestation has occurred.

Semen: Fluid ejaculated consisting of sperm and fluid. This fluid is made by the ducts around the urethra.

Septum: A separation of the uterine cavity.

Super ovulation (super ov): Stimulation of the ovary with drugs in a woman who is already ovulating normally.

Testicular sperm extraction (TESE): Surgical removal of sperm from the testicle.

Testosterone: Male hormone produced by the testicle.

Ultrasonography: An imaging technique that does not use X-ray.

Uterine tube: A tube connected to the uterus that transports the sperm to the egg, picks up the egg from the ovary, where fertilization takes place, and transports the fertilized egg to the uterus.

Varicocele: Dilation of the veins around the testes.

Vas deferens: One of the ducts around the testicle that transports sperm.

ZIFT (zygote intrafallopian transfer): The transfer of the fertilized egg into the tube – usually by laparoscopy.

Index

A

About the Authors

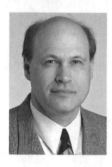

Tommaso Falcone, M.D., is chairman of the Department of Obstetrics & Gynecology at the Cleveland Clinic. He is a graduate of the McGill University Faculty of Medicine in Montreal. Dr. Falcone's specialties include advanced laparoscopic surgery, infertility, in vitro fertilization, microsurgery for tubal ligation reversal, surgery for endometriosis, and infertility surgery.

Davis Young served as a communications advisor to the Cleveland Clinic for more than a decade. He is author of the business management book *Building Your Company's Good Name.* Mr. Young has a special interest in the subject of infertility because of experiences in his own family.

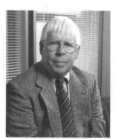

Photo by Mike Wilkes Photography